# THE
# Skinny

THE ULTIMATE GUIDE TO WEIGHT-LOSS SUCCESS

# THE Skinny

## ON
## LOSING WEIGHT WITHOUT BEING HUNGRY

Louis J. Aronne, M.D.,
*with* Alisa Bowman

BROADWAY BOOKS
NEW YORK

Copyright © 2009 by Louis J. Aronne, M.D.

All Rights Reserved

Published in the United States by Broadway Books, an imprint of The Doubleday Publishing Group, a division of Random House, Inc., New York.
www.broadwaybooks.com

BROADWAY BOOKS and its logo, a letter B bisected on the diagonal, are trademarks of Random House, Inc.

Photographs on pp. 119–31 by Beth Bischoff

*Book design by Michael Collica*

Library of Congress Cataloging-in-Publication Data
Aronne, Louis J.
The skinny : on losing weight without being hungry /
Louis J. Aronne : with Alisa Bowman.—1st ed.
            p.      cm.
Includes bibliographical references and index.
1. Weight loss.   2. Reducing diets.   3. Diet.   I. Bowman,
Alisa.   II. Title.
RM222.2.A756 2009
613.2'5—dc22
2008030112

ISBN 978-0-7679-3039-0

PRINTED IN THE UNITED STATES OF AMERICA

2 4 6 8 10 9 7 5 3 1

First Edition

*For my patients,*

*who taught me so much*

*about this area of medicine*

"Dr. Aronne has changed how I think about eating. Food no longer has the power it once did. I don't feel guilty about what I eat and what I don't eat. This has become a way of life."

—*Merri Lee Kingsly, who lost 50 pounds more than 2 years ago*

"Before Dr. Aronne, I walked around feeling like a failure when it came to my weight. I'd been on every diet imaginable, always regaining more than I lost. Now I understand that I didn't have a psychological problem. I had a metabolic problem. This program has been a miracle."

—*Angela McNamee, who lost 70 pounds 1½ years ago*

"One of the big problems with most diets is that big people like me are used to eating a lot of food. Any diet that prescribes small amounts of food is just not going to work. Dr. Aronne's plan did not cut back on the amounts of food I ate, but rather changed the kinds of foods I ate. I was allowed to eat as much of certain types of foods as I wanted."

—*Ryan Elkins, who lost 175 pounds 1½ years ago*

# Contents

## Part Three: Skinny Solutions

## Part Four: Skinny Helpings

# Introduction

Your friends may not believe that you are dedicated to losing weight. Your spouse may not believe you, either. Even your doctor may doubt your sincerity. Well, I believe you. I believe that you want to shed these extra pounds more than you've ever wanted anything, and I believe you are probably willing to do nearly anything to make it happen. In fact, I'd bet a million dollars that if a genie popped out of a little bottle this very moment and granted you just one wish, you would wish for the ability to lose weight.

I believe this because I know just how tremendously difficult—if not impossible—it is to will yourself to eat *less* when your brain keeps telling you to eat *more.*

Why haven't you been able to shrink your portions, forgo dessert, or get yourself to the gym? Why, despite all of your good intentions, do you end up doing the opposite? Why is it that the more you eat, the hungrier you get? These are the very questions I've been studying and trying to answer for the past twenty-three years, ever since Claire came to me for treatment. She was in her late thirties, weighed 270 pounds, and had diabetes, high triglycerides (fat in the blood that tends to clog arteries), and low levels of the health-promoting HDL cholesterol. Her knees were so arthritic that she walked with a cane. I tried *everything* to help her lose weight, and she listened to my every suggestion. We tried, and we tried, and we tried. I studied medical journals. I talked with colleagues. I stayed up late each night thinking about her and why her weight would not budge. I never gave up on her. I didn't, because I knew one thing: there was no way Claire wanted to be that heavy and have those health problems. She wanted to lose weight. She wanted it more than anything. She was miserable in her 270-pound body.

I knew that Claire had to be battling strong biological signals that were driving her to eat. These hormonal signals were obliterating her sense of fullness. I couldn't prove it, but I knew it like I knew the world was round.

Claire's struggle led me, two years later, to develop and found the Comprehensive Weight Control Program at New York Presbyterian Hospital. It was one of the first research and treatment programs in the country devoted to helping people lose weight. My goal was simple: to treat people with weight problems in the same way that our cardiologists treated patients with heart disease. I didn't believe that people with weight problems had psychological or motivational problems. I believed they had a disease, one that could be treated.

To find the best ways to treat this disease, I performed and designed more than twenty-five weight-loss studies, and I consulted with other innovative researchers around the world. I counseled thousands of people, exhaustively working with them to find the most effective eating, behavioral, and lifestyle approaches for lasting weight loss.

I also did media interview after media interview, trying to spread what at the time was an incredibly unpopular message. I wanted people to know that weight loss is *not* about willpower. It's about biology. It's about figuring out why you rarely, if ever, feel full, and about implementing solutions that help you overcome that problem.

Through this research and clinical experience, I've earned a reputation as one of the world's foremost experts in my field. I'm one of the people whom the National Institutes of Health, the Veterans Administration, the American Heart Association, and many others have consulted when they need someone to explain the latest scientific understanding of appetite and metabolism. I'm also the guy folks at CBS News and many other news outlets repeatedly seek out when they want to find out which diets work and which don't. I do multiple television interviews, and countless more for radio and print, all because I want people to know that overeating just isn't their fault.

I'm also the guy to whom physicians from all over the country and world refer their "toughest" patients, the folks who seem destined for weight-loss surgery but who want to give "eating less and moving more" one final try. I see as many as eighty patients every week. They are men and women, celebrities and everyday Joes, adolescents and seniors, executives and clerks. They come from all over the world and are usually somewhere between 50 and 150 pounds overweight. I help many of them drop an average 15 to 20 percent of their initial weight. That's enough to significantly improve their health. That's also the amount of weight they might expect to lose if they opted for lap band surgery. I'm not as proud of the collective pounds they've lost, however, as I am of the sheer numbers of people I've helped, especially the ones, who, without my help, would have otherwise ended up going under the knife.

## The New Skinny on Getting Skinny

When people come to me, they are frustrated. They've been continually trying to shed pounds, yet their weight keeps going up, up, and up. Nearly every day one of them tells me, "I feel like I am losing my mind." They've been insulted and humiliated by well-meaning friends who try to motivate them with tough love. Their family and friends insinuate that they just are not trying hard enough. Their family doctors have read them the riot act, saying things like, "Weight loss is important. If you don't get the weight off, you're going to have a heart attack."

As if they didn't think it was important. As if they were looking forward to having a heart attack. As if they enjoy being overweight in a world that prizes leanness.

During each initial consultation, I start with the question, "Do you feel full when you eat?" It startles patients so much that they often reply, "No one has ever asked me that before." This response doesn't surprise me, in part because I've heard it so many times, but I wish it did. I wish it did because lack of fullness is what prevents so many people from losing weight and keeping it off.

I tell these patients, as I'm now telling you now, that weight loss *isn't* about priorities, willpower, or wanting it badly enough. Rather, it's about biology. It's about your body and your brain and your hormones.

You struggle with your weight because your weight-regulating system is busted. An area of your brain should act as a fuel gauge much like the gas gauge in your car. Instead of measuring the amount of gas in your car, however, it measures the amount of fat and calories in your body. Sensors in your stomach, intestines, and fat cells and elsewhere are supposed to relay messages to your brain, indicating how many calories you've consumed or how much fat is stored in your fat cells. However, these messages aren't getting to your brain, so the needle on your fuel gauge doesn't move and your gauge often reads "empty," even when your stomach is full of food and your fat cells are overflowing with stored calories. The result: you feel hungrier and hungrier, even as you are gaining weight.

Why doesn't your fuel gauge work correctly? The problem may have started when you consumed a diet laden with certain types of foods. It may have begun when you took medications for mood disorders, diabetes, seizures, or other health problems. Not sleeping well or enough, or doing shift work, may have triggered the problem. Whatever the cause, the result is very common, affecting two thirds of the adult population. Children also suffer from the same problem, maybe more than adults. I've treated small children who could eat as much as most adults. Did their parents teach them to eat that much, possibly by placing overly large portions on the table? I don't think so; I believe that a progressive breakdown in the fullness mechanisms ultimately produces this astonishing phenomenon, which I call *feed forward*.

I'd like you to think of this predisposition to gaining weight as a powerful force, as a *health problem* that you must fight. You need a specific set of strategies to override it. If you don't first override the internal biology, typical approaches to weight loss—such as portion control and calorie counting—just don't work. You can't expect to *will* yourself to eat less, stop eating sugar, stop consuming caloric soft drinks, or stop eating bread. You can't, unless you learn how to fix your fullness gauge, so that sensations such as cravings and hunger naturally diminish.

I'll help you fix that gauge with a number of behavioral and eating strategies that have worked time and time again for the men and women I counsel. You'll learn these strategies through a series of incremental steps. Rather than overhauling your diet, joining a gym, and changing many different lifestyle habits at once, you'll be able to focus on small changes, changes such as eating protein for breakfast. Once you make over breakfast, we'll look at lunch. Once you get a handle on lunch, we'll tackle snacks, then dinner, then beverages. Finally, when you are ready, we'll talk about exercise.

These incremental strategies are deceptively simple, so simple that many people hear about them and think, "There's no way *that* works." If you are already feeling a little doubtful, I can't say that I blame you. The weight-loss industry is full of charlatans who want to sell you easy gimmicks. The difference between those gimmicks and my program comes down to one thing: I'm focusing on strategies that will help you do everything you already know you need to do. My strategies do not melt off fat, incinerate calories, or stop you from ever feeling hungry again. They merely take some of the effort out of weight loss, so that you can put down your fork earlier, long before you've overeaten.

I don't believe in false promises. I don't believe in eating and exercise plans that are so hard that you can't possibly follow them. I don't believe in setting you up for failure. I don't believe in lies. I would rather under-promise and overdeliver. I believe in the truth, and the truth is that weight loss is hard. It's hard for everyone, but it's not impossible.

I believe in science, science that says the secret of successful weight loss isn't necessarily about forcing yourself to eat less and exercise more. Rather, it's about learning, understanding, and working with the new science of appetite. That's what *The Skinny* is all about. It's about learning the skinny on why:

- The more you eat of certain foods, the hungrier you seem to get.
- You crave sweets after eating too many carbs.
- You feel cold when you lose weight.
- You wake up feeling hungry after a night of overeating.
- Your metabolism slows as you lose weight.
- You feel hungry after a night of poor sleep.

Most important, I believe in you. I believe that you need not only a program that enables weight loss, but also one you can follow and continue to follow until you lose weight, improve your health, and stay that way for life. Trying to eat less, but can't? Trying to reduce portions, but can't? Trying to cut back on soft drinks, but can't? Welcome to *The Skinny*.

# THE Skinny

# Part One

## The Skinny on Your Appetite

# 1

## The Skinny on Why You Rarely Feel Full

I lecture at Weill-Cornell Medical College in New York City, and invariably, as I explain the physiological underpinnings of appetite, a young man raises his hand. He's usually sitting in a corner in the back of the room. He's slightly built and fit. He's young, and by looking at him I can tell that he's never struggled with his weight a day in his life. Someone just like him sits in that back corner every year. I already know what Naturally Skinny Guy is going to say.

"Yes, you in the back. Do you have a question?" I ask.

"Dr. Aronne," he says, "I understand what you're saying about physiology, but isn't this really about laziness and lack of discipline? Weight loss is really simple. Just push away from the table."

The students chuckle, and some nod their heads in agreement.

"You think it's as easy as just pushing away from the table?" I ask.

"Yes, I do," he says. "To lose weight, people just need to eat less. Just stop eating."

"Okay, if you think it's so easy to push away from the table, I want you to try it. Don't eat until tomorrow's class. I'm putting you on the 24-Hour Water Diet. You can drink all the water you want, but you can't eat anything. Let's see if you can last until tomorrow without eating."

The following morning the medical students file into the lecture hall and take their seats. I ask Naturally Skinny Guy, "How'd it go?" He stares at his shoelaces, so I ask his roommates, "How'd he do?"

"He raided the fridge at three A.M.," they tell me, laughing. "You were right, Dr. Aronne. He couldn't make it."

"Why did you eat?" I ask.

"I didn't feel right. I was so hungry I couldn't sleep."

"Were you able to sleep once you ate?" I ask.

"Yes," he says.

"There, you see," I explain, moving into my lesson, "food has a physiological effect. He thought he knew what to do to lose weight. He thought weight loss was easy. Just don't eat. Where did that advice get him? It got him nowhere. He was so hungry that he couldn't sleep. When overweight people eat less, they often feel just as he described. They don't need to fast for twenty-four hours to feel this way. As soon as they cut back on their calories or portions, they feel lousy and can't function, and when they eat more, they feel better. That's why it's so difficult to lose weight."

## The Appetites of the Naturally Skinny

You may know a few people who think as my med student did. They're the friends and family members who police your grocery cart, restaurant choices, and ice cream bowl. They're the doctors who continually berate you about your weight. They don't understand why you struggle because they've never had to monitor their eating. Naturally skinny people think you're gaining weight because you habitually ignore your body, eating past the sensation of fullness.

"Just listen to your body," these naturally skinny people tell you. "Stop eating when you are full."

"Just halve your portions," they say.

"Stop eating dessert," they tell you.

"Just push away from the table."

These naturally skinny folks are not trying to torment you. They have good intentions, but their advice falls short because they don't understand your eating experience. When these naturally skinny people eat moderate amounts of food, they feel full. They assume everyone does.

For the naturally skinny, the signals that deliver hunger and fullness messages to and from the brain work exquisitely. When a naturally skinny woman sits down to eat, she's hungry. The food in front of her looks and smells delicious. As she chews her first bite, her mouth and stomach register the food's texture and flavor. Excessively sweet flavors tell her brain "high in calories." Bitter foods tell her brain that the food is lower in calories. Thick, heavy liquids—such as a smoothie—tell her brain "high in calories," whereas thin, watery ones—such as fruit juice or water—tell her brain "little to no calories."

As her stomach and intestines fill up with forkfuls of food, these organs secrete a number of signals that travel to her brain. Once she's eaten enough food to fuel cell metabolism for a few hours, these signals trigger fullness. Her stomach feels heavy and distended. Her food tastes and smells bland. Each bite becomes less enjoyable, until, eventually, eating completely loses its pleasure. She puts down her fork and pushes away from the table.

This naturally skinny woman feels full at the exact right moment, when her body no longer needs more calories. She doesn't overeat very often because her brain persuades her not to.

Here's more. When this naturally skinny woman does overeat—say she ignores that sensation of fullness and shovels in some dessert or an extra glass of wine—her brain responds. She feels less hungry at subsequent meals, so she automatically eats less than usual. Her muscles burn more calories to power her every movement, working inefficiently and wasting calories to create body heat. For this naturally skinny woman, the consequence of eating too much is not a larger clothing size or a higher number on the scale. It's that she feels hot when everyone else feels cold. That's why she can stand at the bus stop in the middle of winter without a jacket. Because of these strong, finely tuned, and effective signals, this naturally skinny woman's weight stays fairly constant without dieting, calorie counting, or portion control.

Right about now you probably want to stick a fork in this naturally

**Skinny Mini:** You need only overeat by 10 daily calories to gain 1 pound in one year. That's the amount of calories in two sticks of sugarless gum. (Did you know that sugarless gum has calories? Most people don't.) If you overeat by 100 calories—the calories in a slice of bread or a banana—you'll gain 10 pounds!

skinny woman and everyone like her. I can't say that I blame you. One of my cousins is naturally skinny. She can outeat me and many other men and still fit into a size four. It's frustrating to sit at the same table with her. You may be comforted to know, however, that naturally skinny people are the minority. Fewer than 30 percent of people have skinny genetics; that's why so many of us are overweight.

## The Appetites of Everyone Else

As the naturally skinny woman is pushing away from the table, the rest of us are still eating. We may have consumed the same number of calories as the naturally skinny woman I just described, but we don't feel full. Our food continues to relay fantastic flavors to our brains. Each bite smells and tastes almost as delicious as the first. We don't tire of eating. We may even get hungrier than we felt before the first bite.

Why? The delayed or nonexistent sensation of fullness stems from a condition I call *fullness resistance.* The hormones and chemicals that are supposed to induce fullness no longer work effectively. The fullness signals from the stomach, intestines, and fat cells take longer to reach the brain, and, in some cases, fail to reach the brain at all. In some people fullness *never* kicks in, no matter how much or how often they eat.

You may have been told or believe that overeating stems from a psychological weakness, that it's a way of compensating for stress, frustration, and anxiety. This probably isn't the case. I don't think you are weak. If anything, I believe that you're probably stronger than most people. Day in and day out, you constantly wage

### Do You Have Fullness Resistance?

Answer the following questions with a yes or a no.

1. Have you gained 20 or more pounds since age 20?
2. Do you feel even hungrier after you start eating than you feel on an empty stomach?
3. Do you feel like eating as soon as you get home from eating out?
4. Have you been diagnosed with insulin resistance, pre-diabetes, or type 2 diabetes?

If you answered yes to one or more questions, you could have fullness resistance.

a battle with your brain, with strong physical signals produced during periods of stress, frustration, or anxiety that prompt you hundreds of times a day to eat. You probably find the strength to ignore those nudges to eat *most of the time.*

But you can't expect yourself to be strong enough to wage this type of battle every time you eat. For you, successful weight loss is not about shrinking your portions. It's not about starving yourself. It's not about willpower, and it's probably not about psychology. It's about reversing fullness resistance.

## Your Brain, Your Hormones, and Your Waistline

It may help to think of your body as a car, complete with a gas tank (your stomach and intestines), reserve tank (your fat cells and liver), and a computerized fuel gauge (your brain) that directs you (the driver) to fill these tanks as needed. The needle on your brain's fuel gauge moves based on e-mails (hormones and other chemical messengers) it receives from your main gas tank and reserve tanks, as well as from fuel sensors (your taste buds, your eyes, your nose, and your nerves). Some e-mails flow into the computer with the message "full" and nudge the needle toward the full position. Others come in with the message "empty" and nudge it in the reverse direction.

Brain cells have receptors that function like inboxes for these hunger and fullness e-mails. Some of these cells are clustered together in a hunger center, and others in a fullness center. When hunger hormones reach inboxes on cells in the hunger center, the gauge moves toward the empty position and your stomach rumbles. When fullness hormones reach inboxes on cells in the fullness center, the gauge moves toward the full position and you feel full and satisfied. In experiments done many years ago, researchers damaged the brain's hunger center in rats, shutting down the inbox for hunger hormones. As a result, the fuel gauge was continually in the full position. These rodents never felt hungry. They died from starvation. When researchers instead damaged the fullness center, the rats never felt full. Without a fullness inbox, these rats became obese.

Like those rats, your fullness inbox appears to be broken. The cells in this area of your brain do not activate because they don't receive e-mails from key chemicals and hormones designed to turn off appetite. Fullness hormones fail to nudge the needle on your fuel gauge into the full

**Skinny Mini:** Your body is supposed to give you feedback when you eat. As calories come in, your stomach should eventually feel heavy and distended and thoughts of food should disappear. If you have fullness resistance, however, you don't get feedback. You get *feed forward.* As calories come in, you don't feel full. You feel hungrier sooner, and, when this hunger causes you to overeat, your brain does not turn your appetite down enough or it turns it up, so you overeat between meals or at your next meal.

position. It reads empty, even when your stomach and fat cells are full.

If I gave you a 1982 Buick with a broken fuel gauge, told you I didn't remember the last time I'd filled it with gas, and asked you to drive from New York City to Chicago at midnight, what would you do? You'd stop at every open filling station between New York and Chicago. You'd fill the tank, and once you topped it off, you'd purchase and fill as many extra gas receptacles as you could.

Your brain is treating your body just like that 1982 Buick. It's asking you to continually stop at filling stations (a.k.a. the dinner table, vending machine, pantry, and refrigerator). Once it tops off your main fuel tank (a.k.a. your stomach, gastrointestinal tract, and bloodstream), it opens and fills reserve tanks (a.k.a. your fat cells). It keeps filling more and more fat cells because it doesn't know how much gas it needs or when it will need it.

## Why You're Not Naturally Skinny

Researchers at Laval University in Quebec City, Canada, first uncovered a strong genetic predisposition for weight gain many years ago when they studied twelve sets of identical twins. These twins were all naturally skinny guys in their twenties. Their parents had been skinny, and so had their grandparents. They were as naturally skinny as naturally skinny people can get, but the researchers wanted to see if they could fatten them up.

To do so, the researchers confined these guys inside a college dorm. They forbade them from exercising, and they fed them 1,000 extra calories a day, six days a week for 120 days. That's 84,000 extra calories in 120 days. Given that it takes roughly 3,500 extra calories to gain 1 pound, one would expect that these guys would have gained 23 pounds each. They didn't.

Some sets of twins gained 3½ times more than others, with some gaining as much as 29 pounds and others as little as 9.5 pounds. Yet they all ate the same number of calories. They all lived in the same dorm. They were all equally sedentary.

Why did some of these guys gain so much and others so little? Genes. Each genetically similar twin gained the same amount of weight as his sibling. As it turned out, some of these twins were even more naturally skinny than others. Their bodies resisted weight gain more strongly, turning up their metabolic furnaces and burning an exorbitant amount of calories to produce body heat.

But these guys *were* naturally skinny. Roughly six months after the end of the experiment, they'd all lost the weight they'd gained—naturally.

These researchers have not repeated this experiment by comparing a set of naturally skinny people with a set of natural gainers (it would probably be considered unethical because of the health ramifications), but they have done similar experiments in rats and mice. Rodents genetically engineered with various obesity genes gain more weight than non–genetically altered mice. If a similar experiment were done on people, the natural gainers would gain much more weight than the naturally skinny folks, even if they all consumed the same number of calories.

Thousands of genes are involved in appetite, metabolism, and body weight, and researchers at several institutions have determined that ten times as many of these genes are designed to increase body weight as are designed to decrease it. Known as *thrifty* or *obesity* genes, each of these fat-promoting genes is probably responsible for a small percentage of your propensity to gain weight. You may not have inherited every single obesity gene, but you probably inherited enough of them to raise your risk for gaining weight since before the day you were born.

Depending on which and how many of these genes you inherited from your parents, you may gain weight easily because:

**Skinny Mini:** If both of your parents were overweight, you were born with twice the risk of becoming overweight of someone who was born to naturally skinny parents.

**You have a slow metabolism.** Even if a physician or exercise physiologist has tested your metabolic rate and declared it normal, it may still be slower than it should be. It's difficult to detect differences in metabolic rate because even the smallest of differences—say 10 fewer burned calories a day—can add up to a pound of weight gain in a year. It takes a very small metabolic abnormality to trigger excessive weight gain, and we don't yet have equipment to easily measure the differences that are important.

**You have a heartier appetite.** Could you have fewer "fullness receptors" or inboxes in your brain's fullness center? Fullness hormones can turn off appetite only if they can reach a fullness receptor. If they can't find one, they just circulate throughout the cyberspace of your body, otherwise known as the bloodstream. The result: it takes more calories to shut off your appetite than it does for naturally skinny people.

**Your body stores fat rather than burns it.** Fat cells, like the fullness center of your brain, also have fullness receptors, and when fullness e-mails enter these cells, fat cells release their contents into the bloodstream so muscle cells can burn this fuel for energy. Some people's bodies tend to burn fat rather than store it, whereas other people's bodies tend to store it rather than burn it.

There are many other possible explanations, too. Scientists believe, for example, that the human brain and weight-regulating systems are quite plastic, or changeable, until roughly age 1 and possibly well beyond. Specific experiences during pregnancy and early life may prime the brain for weight gain. If your mother had gestational diabetes, type 1 diabetes, or type 2 diabetes; smoked; drank alcohol; or was overweight or undernourished while she was pregnant with you, you may have been born with a propensity to gain weight. These early life experiences may alter the brain's fullness center, closing off the receptors on important cells and setting you up for fullness resistance. They may have caused your body to maintain a higher number of fat cells, or to have a greater propensity for storing fat rather than burning it.

Such genetics and physiology, by the way, would have come in quite handy a few hundred years ago, when we humans regularly starved for months at a time because of drought and cold winters. Genes that prevent starvation promote obesity. Populations such as the South Seas islanders and southwest U.S. Indians that have gone through the "sieve" of starvation are more likely to be obese. Those with a tendency toward leanness

## The Skinny on . . . Why Undernourished Babies Become Overweight Adults

When scientists tracked the health outcomes of babies born during times of famine, they uncovered an interesting trend. The underweight babies grew into overweight children and adults. During famine, a fetus's leptin levels were low because the mother had less body fat, and this deficiency was probably a protective mechanism, signaling the baby's brain that it would grow up in a world where there isn't much food. Low leptin levels may allow these babies to survive despite malnutrition later in life. The researchers hypothesize that low leptin levels during infancy prevents the fullness center in the brain from developing fully, leading to leptin resistance and a greater tendency toward obesity. Maternal overnutrition and gestational diabetes are just as bad, predisposing babies to developing leptin resistance and obesity, too.

died of starvation, while those with a tendency toward weight gain survived starvation and could pass their genes on to subsequent generations, and these are now the genes that predispose people to obesity.

You are prone to gaining weight just as some people are prone to developing heart disease, breast cancer, and other health problems. It's not your fault. The problem isn't psychological. It's biological.

Once you gain weight, the battle becomes even more difficult. Your body responds to your increasing level of body fat just as it should, by sending fullness messages to your brain in increasing amounts. As these fullness messages flood your brain, however, your brain cells treat them like e-mail spam, putting them on a blocked-senders list. Systems that stimulate hunger, cravings, and the storage of body fat get activated, too. Your brain responds as if you are starving, even though you are overnourished.

As a result, you gain even more weight, which causes the body to produce even more fullness spam and the brain to upgrade its spam filter. Even fewer fullness e-mails reach their intended inboxes, causing a vicious cycle that leads to stronger fullness resistance and more weight gain. It's a one-way trip up the scale.

Your stomach, GI tract, and fat cells secrete a variety of fullness hormones, but the most important of all is leptin. You may have heard of it. I got my first glimpse of its importance in 1986, when my friend and colleague Dr. Rudy Leibel invited me to see very obese mice he was studying, in which the genes for leptin would eventually be discovered. He taught me, and many others, to look at obesity in a completely different way as a result of his novel experiments. In the 1990s pharmaceutical companies thought leptin injections would eventually cure obesity, but, as we later learned, more leptin is not necessarily better.

Here's how leptin works. Your fat cells have internal sensors that tell them when they are filling up. As more fat enters a fat cell, that cell secretes more leptin. Leptin tells your brain's fullness center, "We have enough fuel; don't fill up the gas tank any more." It moves the needle on the gas gauge into the "full" position. Once that happens, other fullness signals can make your stomach feel heavy and reduce the pleasure of eating. With the needle in the "full" position, hunger signals are muffled, too. Consequently, you put down your fork, undo your top button, and push away from the table. If leptin isn't around or the signal isn't received, however, the other signals don't work the way they're supposed to.

The more body fat you have, the higher your leptin levels. Obese people can have up to ten times as much leptin in their blood as naturally skinny people. The increased leptin should amplify the fullness signals, but it doesn't. Obese rats initially respond to leptin injections by losing weight, but after three days the weight loss stops. The excess leptin stops working. Either leptin is not getting to their brains, or their brain cells are not responding to leptin's message. The result: the needle on the gas gauge doesn't move as easily. With the needle in the "empty" position, other fullness hormones become ineffective, too. It takes increasing amounts of fullness hormones to induce the sensation of fullness. Whereas you may once have felt full within just ten minutes of eating a big meal, these signals may now take as long as twenty minutes to induce fullness. The sensation of fullness you do feel is milder than usual, too, so it doesn't always persuade you to stop eating. Eventually, you may still feel hungry even when you've just eaten large quantities of food, or you may never truly feel hungry, but you also never feel full, either, so you continually graze on and on, with no signals to suppress your food intake.

Why does the brain put leptin on a blocked-senders list at all? No one is really sure, but we have some educated theories. According to one of these theories, too much leptin shorts out the system, interrupting the very signaling systems that are needed to listen to and transport the leptin message. It's a fail-safe mechanism, built to encourage you to gain even more weight during periods of feast. In addition, overmetabolism (when the brain turns up metabolism to waste calories as heat) initially caused by overeating generates free radicals, which may damage muscle and brain cells, causing them to be less responsive to leptin and other fullness hormones. In muscles, some of this damage occurs in the mitochondria, the energy-burning compartment of cells. Damaged mitochondria cause muscle cells to burn less fuel, slowing your metabolism and causing more calories to be stored as fat. In the brain, damaged neurons close their doors to leptin, so its message can't get through. Both the brain cells and the muscle cells are shutting down in order to protect themselves from future damage, but you're gaining weight as a result.

Triglycerides, fat in the bloodstream, may also lead to leptin resistance. Researchers at Saint Louis University School of Medicine have shown that triglyceride levels rise along with leptin levels, and triglycerides may act as interference—as an effective spam filter—preventing leptin from reaching the brain. Other factors, including inflammation and high insulin levels, can also lead to leptin resistance.

Interestingly, high leptin levels, the result of leptin resistance, lead to excess inflammation. Leptin has been associated with the inflammation that causes heart disease, as well as other diseases. So elevations of leptin due to leptin resistance, due to obesity, are part of the disease-causing state associated with obesity.

**Skinny Mini:** The number of obese adults increased by 24 percent between 2000 and 2005, with the numbers of the heaviest among us growing the fastest. The number of people with a body mass index, or BMI (a calculation based on weight and height), of more than 40 (about 100 pounds over ideal body weight) increased by 50 percent. The number of those with a BMI of 50 or greater rose by 75 percent. These statistics provide further evidence that some weight gain leads to more weight gain.

One last point about leptin. Some is necessary for normal insulin function. Too little can also cause insulin resistance, in the form of a disorder called *lipodystrophy*. Lipodystrophy can be genetic, or it can be acquired from taking medications for the treatment of HIV infection. In this condition, not enough leptin is present; leptin levels are very low and fat accumulates in the abdomen to compensate. These patients have skinny arms and legs and a big abdomen, with little fat under the skin.

## Insulin: The Fuel Mover

Insulin tells brain cells to signal cells throughout the body to soak up blood sugar and burn it for energy. As blood sugar levels rise, so do insulin levels. Consequently, the more food you eat, particularly carbohydrates, the more insulin your pancreas produces. Because insulin is so instrumental in feeding the hungry cells of your body, it makes sense that this hormone is also responsible for communicating, "Cells are full. No more food needed," to your brain, and that's exactly what it does, assuming all systems are running well.

As with leptin, however, elevated insulin levels cause cells throughout the body to ignore its message. Consuming rapidly digested carbohydrates—sweets, bread, and refined starch—causes blood sugar to rise too quickly, exaggerating the insulin response. If insulin levels remain high or spike to overly high levels consistently, cells throughout your

● ● ● ● ● ● ● ● ● ● ● ● ● ● ● ● ● ● ● ● ● ● ● ● ● ● ● ● ● ● ● ● ● ● ● ● ● ● ● ● ● ● ● ● ● ●

**Skinny Mini:** Most people with insulin resistance don't know it. One unusual symptom is skin problems such as skin tags on the neck, under the arms, or in the breast and groin area. The skin around the neck, knuckles, and elbows also looks dark and velvety, a condition known as *acanthosis nigricans*. If you have these symptoms, mention them to your doctor. I've seen patients who've had dozens of skin tags removed by a dermatologist but were never told that this problem had a possible underlying cause and treatment. People with these skin problems often can't lose weight because their high insulin levels prevent them from making progress, so they need to pair a diet and exercise program with insulin-normalizing medication (see chapter 10).

body and brain put it, as they do with leptin, on a blocked-senders list. When brain cells block insulin's message, this hormone rises in the blood but does not reach the brain. It screams, "Way too much energy in the body," but the brain doesn't hear the message.

When muscle cells stop listening to insulin, they stop burning as much fuel. Your metabolism slows, less blood sugar is burned, and insulin triggers the liver to convert sugar into triglycerides, which are stored in your fat cells and contribute to leptin and even greater insulin resistance. As you can see, it's a vicious cycle, a feed-forward mechanism that leads to greater levels of obesity.

## Other Fullness Chemicals

You don't need to remember the names of the following hormones. You certainly don't need to know how to spell them, or even remember where they are made or what they do. Just remember that many hormones are designed to make you feel full, but you don't feel full because one or several of them are not working effectively. The reason: when leptin is on the blocked e-mail list, some of these signals such as CCK and GLP-1 are not received properly by the brain, leading to a diminished sense of fullness.

**Dopamine:** This brain chemical triggers the sensation of pleasure. Levels rise dramatically when you eat high-calorie, sweet, fatty foods, rewarding you for these food choices and making you feel better. Researchers from Brookhaven National Laboratory in Upton, New York, have determined that obese people may have fewer dopamine receptors (or inboxes). Possibly a result of chronic stress, the reduced number of receptors may cause a person to eat more sugary or starchy foods to raise dopamine levels high enough and often enough to induce the pleasurable feeling that naturally skinny people can get by eating much less food. This is one reason why it's so important to exercise, because physical activity may activate dopamine receptors, reducing cravings and allowing you to feel satisfied with less.

**Cholecystokinin (CCK):** Released from the GI tract after meals, CCK stimulates the release of digestive juices, slows stomach emptying, and suppresses appetite. If you are leptin resistant, CCK may not produce as much fullness as it should.

**Glucagon-like peptide (GLP-1):** Made in the intestine, glucagon-like peptide rises as you eat to induce fullness. You may produce less of this hormone than you need, and you may also be resistant to amounts you do produce.

**Peptide YY:** Blood levels of this peptide drop before meals, causing your stomach to rumble. The levels rise as you eat and, along with GLP-1, help induce fullness. In one study, peptide YY did not rise as much in obese study participants as it did in thinner participants who consumed the same amount of food.

## The Hunger Hormones

Three major hunger hormones set naturally skinny people apart from everyone else.

**Endocannabinoids (ECs):** Notice that the second half of this word resembles a chemical you may have learned about in tenth-grade health class. ECs are similar to cannabis, the chemical found in marijuana. Since at least A.D. 300, cannabis has been known to stimulate hunger and increase appetite, especially for sweets. ECs do the same thing.

When ECs rise, you feel hungry, particularly for sweets. Naturally skinny people probably don't have as intense cravings for sweets because their EC levels are lower than yours, and their brains don't listen as closely to the ECs that are floating around. They are sensitive enough to the leptin sent to their brains by their fat cells to block the action of ECs.

As you gain weight, ECs rise and strengthen. Without enough leptin signaling in the brain to block their signals, EC messages can come into your brain's hunger inbox with "high priority" exclamation points. As a result, you feel hungry when you should feel full, and you crave foods that are loaded with fat and sugar. Think chocolate. Think pie. Think ice cream. Thanks to ECs, you eat more and more often, gain weight, and burn fewer calories. This is an example of the feed-forward mechanism that's leading to the epidemic of obesity in our country and around the world. Once you start eating unhealthy foods, systems such as the ECs feed forward, increasing your appetite and reducing your satiety. The more often you consume sweet, fatty foods or starchy, fatty foods, the hungrier you feel. Sound familiar? I bet it does. It drives you crazy because you know you're supposed to feel full and stop eating, but you don't. The result is the problem some call *gluttony*. It's not a behavioral problem; it's a physical problem that's induced by poor eating choices and worsened by genetically encoded physiology. If you try to change your behavior by eating differently, your body resists your efforts, limiting your ability to succeed at weight loss.

High EC levels also signal other organs in the body. For example, they tell the liver to convert blood glucose into triglycerides and store those triglycerides in fat cells. In your muscles, ECs inhibit the effects of insulin, causing insulin levels to rise even more. In your fat cells, they suppress release of adiponectin, the result of which is even greater resistance to insulin. In the pancreas, ECs inhibit production of insulin, predisposing you to high blood glucose.

● ● ● ● ● ● ● ● ● ● ● ● ● ● ● ● ● ● ● ● ● ● ● ● ● ● ● ● ● ● ● ● ● ● ● ● ● ● ● ● ● ● ● ●

### The Skinny on . . . Why Dieting Makes You Feel Cold

Walk into any weight-loss surgery center in the middle of summer and check out what the bariatric patients are wearing. Many are wearing sweaters even though it's hot and humid. Why?

Many people expect overweight people to feel hot because they assume that the excess fat insulates the body. Although this is true to some extent, body heat is determined more by food intake and levels of certain hormones than by body fat levels, just as the ambient temperature of your home is determined more by the output of your heater than it is by the insulation in your walls. Flip off the heater in the middle of winter and no amount of insulation will keep the house warm. The same happens when you go on a diet.

Less food is coming in and fat cells are shrinking. Leptin levels are dropping. As leptin levels drop, your metabolism and thyroid function slow, and your muscles don't produce as much heat, so you feel cold. This coldness is also an appetite trigger, encouraging you to eat.

Taking supplemental thyroid hormone isn't the solution, as an underactive thyroid isn't the true problem. Low leptin levels are. Exercise, on the other hand, does seem to help. It builds muscle, which creates body heat. By exercising, you prevent your muscles from being able to compensate for the reduction in calories, body weight, and leptin, helping also to normalize thyroid function.

**Ghrelin:** Made in the stomach and intestines, ghrelin rises just before meals and then drops as you eat. This hunger hormone may stay elevated for a longer period of time after you eat than it does for naturally skinny people. One study found that normal-weight people experienced a 39 percent drop in ghrelin within thirty minutes after eating. In obese people, there was no drop during this time. When you lose weight, ghrelin levels increase. That's part of the reason you may go off your diet.

**Cortisol:** Chronic stress has been shown to promote the release of cortisol from the adrenal gland and increase cravings for comfort foods. In turn, the consumption of comfort foods reduces the perception of stress in rats. That explains why foods like cookies and chocolate are so comforting. They really do seem to reduce the perception of stress and anxiety! To make matters worse, feeding efficiency—the number of calories the body stores after you eat—is also increased when you are under chronic stress, leading to an increased likelihood of gaining weight. Finally, increased cortisol levels produce insulin resistance and the accumulation of fat in the abdomen, the riskiest fat to have.

## Then You Reach a Plateau

Our bodies are programmed to resist weight loss that goes beyond roughly 7 percent of total body weight, more or less depending on the person. That means if you weigh 150 pounds, you may be able to lose fewer than 11 pounds before the going gets tough. This is a survival mechanism designed to prevent starvation, but it's frustratingly inconvenient if you weigh 250 pounds and want to weigh 150 pounds instead.

Weight loss causes muscle cells to become more efficient. It's similar to a big gas-guzzling SUV getting better gas mileage as the gas gauge moves closer to the "empty" position. (Perhaps an executive at an automotive company will read this book and decide to invent such a vehicle!) Like the SUV I just described, as your fuel levels drop, your body gets more "miles per gallon" from the food you eat and the fat you have stored. Your body burns fewer and fewer calories as you eat fewer and fewer calories.

Leptin levels will be low, too, so you'll lose your sense of fullness and feel hungry all the time. You're trapped between that quintessential rock and a hard place. In this case, the rock is a more efficient metabolism and the hard place is hunger and cravings that force you to eat. Even if you can ignore the hunger and stick to your diet, you plateau anyway because your metabolism slows.

So how do you get past a plateau? You have to follow the right type of diet, and you have to do the right types of exercise. The low-glycemic diet and exercise plan in this book will help by improving insulin sensitivity. When insulin levels normalize, leptin sensitivity improves, and all of a sudden the weight-regulating mechanism becomes "competent" again, receiving the e-mail messages from the fat cells appropriately

## The Skinny on . . . Why Food Tastes Better When You're Dieting

Back in the 1980s and 1990s we used to recommend a low-calorie liquid diet. For three months patients would drink five shakes a day, shakes that nourished them with just 800 daily calories. Most humans consume about 2,000 calories a day to maintain their weight, so 800 calories is very little.

After these patients reached their goal, they would typically have chicken breast and vegetables as their first solid meal. It's not a particularly tasty or exciting meal, and that was exactly the point. The somewhat bland meal was designed to prevent these patients from experiencing a culinary nirvana that triggered over-eating. Yet my patients consistently reported that the chicken was the best chicken they'd ever tasted. They'd come to me the week after introducing this meal and say things like, "I don't know where I got that chicken, but it was the juiciest, most delicious chicken I've ever had."

I knew better. The chicken wasn't special. It wasn't any more juicy or flavorful than chicken they'd had any number of times throughout their lives. The difference now was that their senses were heightened. High ECs, low leptin, and many other mechanisms primed their taste buds and nose to deliver sensational messages to their brains about the chicken's taste and smell. Their subsequent meals of chicken or almost anything else would never come close to that initial thrill.

rather than blocking them and, as a result, reducing hunger and cravings and increasing metabolism.

## Fix the Fullness Gauge

In the following pages, I will reveal an exciting program designed to help you reverse fullness resistance, lose weight, and keep it off for life. In the next chapter, you'll learn about the newest science-based approaches to eating that help fix the underlying brain chemistry that contributes to overeating. Then I'm going to teach you how to be satisfied with less. I'll teach you how to automatically put down your fork and push away from the table without counting a single calorie.

# 2

# The Skinny on Fattening Foods and Filling Foods

You need lose only 5 to 10 percent of your weight to reverse full-ness resistance. That's just 10 pounds if you weigh 200. The prob-lem is that those 10 pounds can feel like 1,000 pounds if you use the wrong eating approach. On this plan, your first 10 pounds will feel like 10 pounds—and not like a hundred or a thousand—because you'll be consuming the world's most satisfying and filling foods. These satisfy-ing foods allow you to eat three-course meals, complete with a glass of wine if you desire. You'll lose weight by eating more.

By consuming the world's most filling foods, you'll stop eating before you've overeaten. A University of Sydney review of many different diets concluded that the type of eating approach showcased in this book results in just as much weight loss as calorie-controlled diets—if not more—even if study participants ate as much as they wanted, without restricting portions.

# What Are Fattening Foods?

To understand how this works, let's define a couple of terms. First, let's talk about the word *fattening*. When you think of a fattening food, what comes to mind? Most people think of chocolate cake, cookies, and brownies. Those foods *are* fattening, but probably not for the reasons that you think. Most people think these foods are fattening because they are rich in calories.

I'd like to introduce you to a new understanding of fattening foods. Fattening foods are fattening because they trigger cravings or rebound hunger. Foods are fattening when they break your fuel gauge, telling the brain that you have not eaten as much as you have, setting off your feed-forward mechanisms. By that definition, bagels can be fattening. So can low-fat muffins. So is fruit juice. Diet soft drinks may be fattening, too.

Fattening foods generally contain one or more of the following ingredients or characteristics: rapidly digested carbohydrate, high amounts of dietary fat, sugar, or empty calories. In the following pages, I'll explain why each of those characteristics tends to trigger weight gain.

**Rapidly digested carbohydrate is fattening.** Carbohydrate is the sugar, starch, and fiber found in plant foods. The GI tract breaks down the carbohydrate you eat into sugar for your cells to either burn for en-

. . . . . . . . . . . . . . . . . . . . . . . . . . . . . . . . . . . . . . . . . .

## The Skinny on . . . Why You Feel Hungrier after You Start Eating

Many of my patients tell me that they do just fine between meals. It's once they start eating that things really go awry. "Dr. Aronne," they tell me, "I'm not hungry until I eat. I plan to eat only a little bit, but once I start eating, I get hungry. The more I eat, the hungrier I get."

What's going on? They feel hungrier because they're consuming rapidly digested carbohydrates. These foods dramatically raise blood sugar, resulting in an insulin surge that quickly drives sugar back down, causing rebound hunger. This happens only if you eat hunger-promoting foods. If you consume filling foods—such as the ones on the *Skinny* menus—hunger will dissipate with each forkful, and you'll fill up rather than fill out.

ergy or store for later use. As the GI tract breaks down carbohydrate and allows this sugar to enter the bloodstream, the pancreas produces insulin to shuttle sugar into body cells. The more slowly the GI tract breaks down a high-carbohydrate food, the more gradual the rise in blood sugar, and the more gradual the rise in insulin. The more quickly the GI tract breaks down carbohydrate, the faster and more dramatic the rise in blood sugar, and the more dramatic the rise in insulin.

If you consume too much rapidly digested carbohydrate at once, insulin levels rise too high and drive down blood sugar levels too quickly, leading to rebound hunger and interfering with the leptin-signaling mechanism, leading to leptin resistance. Another gut hormone called glucose-dependent insulinotropic peptide (GIP) also rises when you consume starch, and it rises faster and more dramatically when you consume rapidly digested starch. This gut hormone is responsible for gauging when starch comes in too quickly for body cells to burn. High levels of GIP flip a fat-storage switch. They start the conversion of starch into triglycerides (fat) and signal fat cells to soak up this fat from the bloodstream.

One way to reverse fullness resistance, reduce hunger, and discourage fat storage is to consume carbohydrate foods that result in slow and gradual rises in both insulin and GIP. These foods are all low in glycemic load (GL), which is a measure of how quickly food raises blood sugar levels. Foods with high GL raise blood sugar more quickly than foods with low GL. The more quickly blood sugar rises, the more quickly insulin and GIP rise, too.

In a Boston Children's Hospital study of seventy-three overweight teens, those who followed a low-GL diet improved insulin sensitivity and lost more weight and body fat than teens who followed a low-fat diet, especially if they had insulin resistance before the study began. In another study done at the same hospital, overweight adults who followed a low-GL diet experienced a less severe drop in energy expenditure, or metabolism, with weight loss compared to those who ate a low-fat diet. Participants on the low-GL diet also reported less hunger, and their insulin resistance, triglycerides, C-reactive protein (a measure of inflammation and risk factor for heart disease), and blood pressure improved more than for study participants who consumed a low-fat diet. All in all, a low-GL diet looks like the best approach for most people.

How do you know whether a food is high or low in GL? In chapter 13,

I've listed the GL for dozens of commonly consumed foods, but there are three easy ways to tell.

1. Low-GL foods are low in starch and sugar. The more starch or sugar a food contains, the more raw material the GI tract has to convert into blood sugar. For this reason, most legumes and vegetables—with the exception of some types of root vegetables—are all low in glycemic load. An entire head of Boston Bibb lettuce, for example, contains fewer than 4 grams of carbohydrate and 16 calories. Compare that to a slice of bread, which has roughly 16 grams of carbohydrate and 90 calories.

2. Low-GL foods tend to be high in fiber. This nondigestible form of carbohydrate slows the absorption of sugar into the bloodstream and reduces the glycemic load of a high-carbohydrate food.

3. Low-GL foods are whole foods. Foods made from sugar or refined flour—white rice, white bread, snack chips, and sweets—are universally high in GL. Most whole foods— vegetables, legumes, and whole grains—are medium to low in GL.

**Calorie-dense foods are fattening.** Calorie-dense foods contain a lot of calories per bite. Because such foods pack so many calories into a small amount of space, it's easy to eat thousands of calories of such foods and not remotely feel satisfied. For example, chocolate kisses are calorie-dense. Just eight of these mini-candies add up to 200 calories but do very little to fill you up. On the other hand, you would have to eat several bell peppers—which have a very low calorie density—to total the same amount of calories. Calorie-dense foods are usually high in fat or sugar (or both) and low in water and fiber.

**Dietary fat is fattening.** For many years, an unfortunate and misguided debate has stymied nutrition experts. On one side of this debate stood staunch believers in low-fat diets who claimed that fat was fattening. On the other side were the believers in high-fat or high-protein diets who claimed that carbohydrate was fattening.

Who's right? Neither side. As it turns out, both can be fattening, for different reasons.

Fat contains 9 calories per gram compared to just 4 calories per gram for carbohydrate and protein. That means that foods that are high in fat also contain a lot of calories, and these calories are often packed into a small amount of space. Consider that the calories in a 12-ounce portion of prime rib—one of the fattiest cuts of red meat—total more than 1,000. Compare that to the calories in the same-size portion of skinless chicken breast: 512. You'd have to consume nearly 24 ounces of chicken to total the 1,000 calories in the 12-ounce prime rib. I don't know too many people who can eat that much chicken without feeling uncomfortably full, but I know plenty of people, myself included, who can consume a 12-ounce steak. For this reason, it's extremely easy and tempting to overeat high-fat foods.

Fat may be fattening for a few additional reasons. Fatty foods do not suppress the hunger hormone ghrelin as quickly or as much as protein does, and research done at the University of Leeds suggests that they may not suppress hunger at all. Study participants ate either 350 excess calories of carbohydrate or 350 excess calories of fat for breakfast and then monitored their hunger and eating for the rest of the day. The carbohydrate eaters compensated by eating about 350 calories less for lunch and dinner. The fat eaters didn't eat less later on. The fat came in under their brain's caloric radar. It didn't move the fuel gauge. They continued to eat as they normally would and ended their days with a 350-calorie surplus.

The *trans fats* (also called *hydrogenated fats*) in margarine and processed foods and the *saturated fats* in

The Skinny on . . .
Whether Dietary Fat
Slows Digestion
Some diets encourage you to add fat to quickly digested starch to reduce the speed at which the starch enters the bloodstream and raises blood sugar. For example, if you're going to have a baked potato, these diets urge, have it with sour cream or butter. Although this tactic does reduce GL, it backfires in other ways. The combination of sugar or starch with fat tends to trigger the body to store these excess calories as fat, rather than burn them for energy. It also may result in rebound hunger or cravings for similar high-calorie foods. In rat studies, increases in saturated fat consumption led to insulin and leptin resistance.

## The Skinny on . . . Why Heavy Foods Lead to Light Appetites

The fullness hormones of naturally skinny people seem to respond equally effectively to both the weight and the caloric content of the food they eat. When a naturally skinny person consumes a calorie-loaded food—such as a fast-food burger—that is small in size and light in weight, she still feels full and stops eating, sometimes midburger. Your fullness hormones, however, may respond more quickly and effectively to the weight and volume of your food than they do to the caloric content of your food. Low-volume, lightweight, high-calorie foods such as French fries, soft drinks, and candy bars leave you feeling hungry, even though you've consumed many more calories than your body needs. High-volume, low-calorie, low-fat foods that weigh a lot such as salad, vegetables, lean protein, and legumes fill you up, because they more quickly and effectively trigger the release of fullness hormones.

- - - - - - - - - - - - - - - - - - - - - - - - - - - - - - - - - - - - - - - - -

fatty animal products (whole milk, cheese, fatty cuts of meat, chicken skin) may be particularly problematic because they may raise levels of triglycerides and contribute to inflammation, both of which lead to fullness resistance. In fact, some research indicates that mothers who consume diets rich in trans fats during pregnancy give birth to children with a higher risk of developing insulin resistance.

Are you worried that you'll miss the taste of fat? Don't be. *Skinny* recipes will show you easy ways to shrink fat without losing out on flavor, and research shows that most people get used to low-fat eating and just stop thinking about it. In a Penn State study of more than 250 women, women who cut fat to lose weight eventually reduced their palatability rankings of high-fat foods. They lost their "fat tooth."

**Sugar is fattening.** Sugar is a type of rapidly digested carbohydrate, and for many people it's addictive. Rats, for example, experience withdrawal symptoms, including a drop in body temperature and aggression, when sugar is added to their diet and then removed.

For many years, scientists speculated that cane sugar was less harmful than high-fructose corn syrup, a sweetener made from corn starch. As it

## The Skinny on . . . Why You Feel Hungry an Hour or Two after Eating a Bagel

Most bagels contain somewhere between 300 and 400 calories. That amount of calories should, theoretically, hold you over until lunch. Why doesn't it? Bagels are high in carbohydrate. This macronutrient suppresses the hunger hormone ghrelin quickly, causing you to feel satisfied just after eating. The problem is, however, that high-carbohydrate meals tend to trigger a rebound effect. They drive down ghrelin initially, but this hormone then rises to higher-than-normal levels within just a few hours, causing you to feel even hungrier than you did before you ate. Protein foods, such as eggs, don't suppress this hormone as quickly as carbohydrate foods, but they suppress it for a longer period of time. This is why you may still feel hungry immediately after finishing an omelet, but then eventually feel satisfied, a sensation that lasts for many hours.

If you do feel full until lunch when you have a bagel with cream cheese for breakfast, it's probably because you're eating a super-large bagel. Check out the number of calories. I bet it's approaching 700! If you want to try the carb-vs.-protein experiment yourself, make sure you eat the same number of calories of carbohydrate and protein foods. I bet the protein foods hold you longer.

turns out, it probably doesn't matter what form of added sugar is in your food or beverage. Cane sugar and high-fructose corn syrup are probably equally fattening because of the sheer numbers of excess calories they provide and their excessive sweetness. Artificial sweeteners may also be problematic. Their excessive sweetness may cause you to continually crave other sweet foods such as cookies. Some researchers also believe that artificial sweeteners may disrupt how the brain senses the calories in your food. The brain associates sweet flavors with calories, but artificial sweeteners are both sweet and low in calories. Rats alternatively given water sweetened with either sugar or an artificial sweetener ate more chow than rats given only sugar water or plain water. The artificially sweetened water seemed to prime their brains with an inconsistent message, preventing their brains from correctly monitoring their calorie intake.

**Empty calories are fattening.** Our bodies evolved on foods that nourished us with more than just calories. The vegetables, legumes, game meat, and fruit our ancient ancestors consumed were rich in vitamins, minerals, and many other nutrients that our bodies need to perform countless chemical reactions. When you consume a diet rich in junk foods such as potato chips, cheese doodles, and dessert, you consume a diet that is poor in nutrition. Theoretically, cells starved for specific nutrients may signal your brain to turn up your appetite, causing you to eat until those nutrient needs are met.

## What Are Filling Foods?

*The Skinny* eating plans use every scientific finding to help you fill up on fewer calories. You will fill every plate with low-calorie, low-GL foods that are rich in appetite-suppressing fiber, protein, and water. Filling foods feature one or more of the following nutrients or characteristics.

**Lean protein is filling.** *The Skinny* meal makeovers include lean protein at every eating opportunity. Various studies on animals and humans show that protein induces fullness faster than fat and for longer than carbohydrate. When men consumed a high-protein yogurt as part of a study done at Adelaide Hospital in Australia, they ate 9 percent less at subsequent meals than they did after consuming a high-fat yogurt and 12 percent less than after eating a high-carbohydrate yogurt.

Research completed at Arizona State University shows that protein-rich meals also kick up your metabolism for as long as 2.5 hours after eating. Protein foods enable the leptin message to more easily reach important brain cells that literally turn up the heat—by raising body temperature—on your metabolism. High-protein meals, these researchers found, produce two times as much calorie burning during this post-meal window as high-carbohydrate meals do.

**Low-calorie foods are filling.** Low-calorie foods contain few calories per bite. They are rich in water and low in fat and sugar. Think fruits, vegetables, soup, and salad. You can fill up with a hearty portion of these foods—thanks to their low calorie density—but consume very few calories in the process. One study done by Barbara Rolls, Ph.D., and her colleagues at Penn State determined that switching from a diet composed of foods with a high calorie density to one primarily composed of foods with a low calorie density allowed seventy-one women to naturally consume fewer calories—without actually counting calories or watching portion sizes. These women also lost more weight over six months than did a different group of dieters who reduced fat but did not reduce calorie density.

**Wholesome foods are filling.** *The Skinny* menus feature vegetables, legumes, and many other highly nutritious foods to nourish cells throughout your body with the vitamins, minerals, and nutrients they need. I can't prove that wholesome foods turn down appetite, but it makes sense in theory, and some research seems to support the concept. For example, a Bastyr University Research Institute study of more than 15,000 men and women determined that study participants who took a multivitamin gained less weight during ten years than participants who did not use a multivitamin.

**Heavy, high-volume foods are filling.** *The Skinny* menus feature foods that are relatively heavy in weight and high in volume, but low in calories. These foods—such as soup, vegetables, fruit, and salad—weigh down your stomach, signaling stretch receptors in your stomach and intestines to tell your brain, "I'm full."

**Slow foods are filling.** Slow foods take a long time to eat or a long time to digest, or both. As you gain weight, it takes longer for the "I'm full" message to reach your brain. This is why you've probably heard that you should eat slowly; it allows this all-important message to reach the brain. Here's the problem with that advice. Who can do it? I've tried to eat slowly, and I can tell you, it's difficult. We all have a natural eating pace, and, although I encourage you to try to slow down, I also have a more effective solution for this problem. By eating "slow" foods first—chewy, crunchy, or heavy, watery foods such as soup, salad, and vegetables—you will *automatically* consume your calories more slowly. It's unbelievably easy to slurp down hundreds of calories from starchy, fatty foods in record time. Think about how quickly you could eat 500 calories of fettuccine alfredo (roughly a third of the portion you'd be served at most restaurants). Five minutes? Now, think about how long it would take for you to eat 500 calories of shrimp cocktail. That's 67 large shrimp. Even if they came prepeeled, you would be sitting at the table for quite a while.

I hope you now understand that weight loss does not have to be about counting calories, because a calorie is not a calorie. You could eat

500 calories of chicken and broccoli or 500 calories of cookies, but the chicken and broccoli will fill you up and the cookies will fill you out, and you'll become hungrier sooner after eating them.

## Fattening vs. Filling Foods

What makes some foods fattening and others filling?
Use this cheat sheet.

| Fattening | Filling | Why? |
|---|---|---|
| High-fat dairy and meat products | Lean dairy and meat | Protein induces long-lasting fullness, but fat does not. Remove the fat and you induce fullness with fewer calories. |
| Sweet flavors | Spicy flavors | Sweet flavors may be addictive. Spicy, bitter, and other flavors from capsaicin, cinnamon, and other herbs and spices increase the joy of eating without causing overeating. |
| Thin liquids (fruit juice, soft drinks, and other sources of liquid calories) | Thick liquids (chunky soup, smoothies, and other viscous foods and beverages) | Thin liquids escape your body's caloric radar. Calories come in, but the needle on your fuel gauge never moves. Thick liquids stimulate nerves in the stomach and intestines that help move the needle to the full position. |
| Foods made from refined flour | Vegetables, fruit, legumes, and whole grains | Refined flour is both devoid of nutrition and high in rapidly digested carbohydrate, both of which induce hunger. Vegetables, fruit, legumes, and other whole foods are rich in water, are heavy, take a long time to eat, and are rich in fiber, all of which help fill you up. |

| Fattening | Filling | Why? |
| --- | --- | --- |
| Pasta, bread, and other high-carbohydrate foods | Lean animal protein | Protein induces long-lasting fullness. Pasta and other carbohydrate foods may induce fullness initially, but often lead to rebound hunger. |

## Eat Filling Foods First and Fattening Foods Last

Most diets tell you what you can't eat. What happens when you think about what you can't eat? You want to eat the food you're trying not to eat, right? I believe that successful weight loss is a matter of addition, not subtraction. Instead of thinking about all of the fattening foods you are trying not to eat, I'd rather you focused on all of the filling foods you are trying *to* eat.

Don't tell yourself that you are not allowed to have bread, wine, or dessert. You can have these foods if you really want them, but you just have to consume filling foods *first*. If you absolutely, positively will not feel complete unless you've had a piece of chocolate or a scoop of ice cream, have it, but only have it shortly after dinner. If you follow this one rule, you will automatically consume fewer fattening foods without really thinking about it.

Let's take bread as an example. We all love it, right? Yet bread is a hunger-promoting food. It digests quickly, is relatively light, and provides very little staying power per calorie consumed. Case in point: most people could polish off five or six crusty dinner rolls at a restaurant and still have room for an appetizer and main course, even though those rolls set them back roughly 600 calories! If I told you that you could never eat bread again, however, what would happen? You'd start thinking about bread, wouldn't you? At first, these thoughts might not be too bothersome. Over a period of days, however, they would grow stronger and stronger until you could not stop thinking about bread. You'd probably dream about it, too. Then, what do you think would happen when you inevitably go out to eat at a restaurant that brings warm rolls to the table as soon as you sit down? You would eat everything in the basket, right? I'm pretty sure that's what I'd do.

Now think about this. What if, instead of telling you that you could never have bread or sugar or beer or any other fattening food again, I told you that you could have these foods, but you had to earn them by eating filling foods first? You could have the bread, but you first had to eat a salad and then a plate of steamed vegetables followed by chicken or fish. What do you think would happen? My patients tell me that they feel so satisfied that either they don't want the bread or they eat just one small serving and feel satisfied.

Isn't that a more pleasant way to lose weight? I sure think so, and so do the thousands of patients I've counseled. Throughout the pages of *The Skinny,* you'll learn many strategies like the one I just described that will help you automatically eat less of many different fattening foods and beverages: soft drinks, dessert, and more.

# 3

# The Skinny on How to Follow
## *The Skinny*

In the following pages, you'll find important advice for following the plan. You'll also find the basic eating plan that I give to my patients. You have a choice. You can incorporate all of the eating and lifestyle changes at once, as they are outlined in this chapter, or you can take them one change at a time. Chapters 4–9 will walk you through this step-by-step approach.

Which approach is better? That depends on you. To decide, think about the following questions:

**Are you the type of person who feels energized by the thought of wholesale dietary and lifestyle changes?** If you answered yes, then you can transition to *The Skinny*'s eating and exercise plans as soon as today. I've laid out all of the nutritional principles you'll need in this chapter, but I encourage you to read chapters 4–9, too. These chapters provide a more detailed rationale behind the food choices. If you understand why the plan works, you'll more easily be able to get yourself to follow it. These chapters also include a lot of helpful advice, such as how to get yourself to eat breakfast when you are not hungry in the morning.

**Are you the type of person who feels intimidated by huge dietary and lifestyle changes?** In other words, are you already forming excuses in your mind for why you can't possibly stick with this or any other weight-loss plan? If you answered yes, then I encourage you to tackle the plan one step at a time. Read this chapter to understand the basic structure of the plan, and then turn to chapter 4 to learn more about your first dietary change: breakfast. Get used to eating the right types and amounts of foods for breakfast; once that feels habitual, move on to lunch, then dinner, then snacks, and then beverages. Spend at least a week with each dietary change before tackling the next. This step-by-step approach has worked well for my patients. That's why I know it can work for you.

Many people ask me why I don't encourage exercise from day one. If you love to exercise and are already exercising, don't stop. By all means, keep it up. If you're raring to go, go ahead, but if you hate exercise, as many of my patients do, there's no reason to grit your teeth through it from day one. Your dietary habits play a larger role in managing fullness resistance and in helping you to lose weight than your exercise habits do. You can start to reverse fullness resistance with food alone, without taking a single extra step of lifting one dumbbell. Each incremental dietary change you make on this plan will help you make the next step. Changing breakfast will turn down hunger at lunch. Making over lunch reduces hunger and cravings at dinner. Making over your meals and snacks will help you more easily give up sugary soft drinks. Once you do all of that, you'll have more energy, so exercise will feel easier. Besides improving your health, the role of exercise is to lower your plateau and help you maintain, two factors that become more important once you've already lost some weight.

## Before You Start

My nutrition and exercise plans are designed to help you reduce hunger on a physiological level. I'd be remiss, however, if I did not give you a few tools to help you stick with these plans on a psychological level. In my opinion, you don't have a psychological problem, but psychological tools can be used to help you to succeed. Before you change one meal, I encourage you to do the following:

**1. Commit to the program.** You should be able to answer the following questions with a resounding "Yes!" If you answer no to any of these questions, this may not be the best time for you to try to lose weight. Ideally, start the program at a time that allows you to commit to many months of hard work.

- Are you ready to make an effort to change your lifestyle permanently?
- Do you have nonvanity-related reasons for wanting to lose weight (better health, more energy, less pain, more self-esteem)?
- Do you have time to commit to weight loss?
- Are you free of commitments (holidays, job promotion, care of a new child) that may hinder your ability to focus on changing your lifestyle?
- Is keeping the weight off long term more important to you than initial short-term losses?

**2. Keep a lifestyle log.** Many studies show that people who keep a weight-loss diary lose up to twice as much weight as people who do not, and dieters who write down what they eat are also more likely to keep off what they lose. Your food and exercise journal can help you do the following:

- Pinpoint barriers to weight loss. For example, many people don't consciously notice those little nibbles of food—those bites you sampled from your child's plate of macaroni and cheese, for example. When you write down what you eat as soon as you eat it, you'll more likely notice these little nibbles, which allows you to take steps to follow the plan more precisely in the future.
- Determine *why* you eat certain foods. For instance, if you jot down your mood, stress level, or hunger level along with what you ate, you will be able to look at your journal and see if you ate a particular food because you felt stressed, were sad, or were celebrating.
- Stay accountable to your goals. Many people have a harder time cheating on their nutritional goals when they know they have to write down what they eat.

Plus, keeping a journal is cheap and easy and has no side effects. I don't require you to keep a specific type of journal; I only recommend that you write something down every day. You can keep a detailed log, or you can just capture rough notes. Do what works best for you. You can keep it on your PalmPilot, on your cell phone, or in a little notebook that you carry around with you.

Consider keeping track of the following:

- **What you eat:** Carry your journal with you and write down everything you eat and drink. Include the time you ate it, along with what else you were doing or feeling. Whenever you cheat, jot down some notes about why you ate what you did, whether you could have chosen a better food, and whether you ate because you were hungry. These clues may help you later in coming up with ways to avoid nibbling on those same foods in the future.
- **How hungry you feel:** Before eating, rate your hunger on a scale of 1 to 10, with 10 so ravenous you could eat your foot and 1 being almost full. If your number is less than a 5, don't eat.
- **Your lifestyle activity:** As you incorporate more lifestyle activity, jot down each incremental step in the right direction, such as the first time you walked into the bank rather than used the drive-through. You'll find specific advice for incorporating more lifestyle activity in chapter 9.
- **Your mood:** Write down how you feel when you eat, especially if you find yourself eating starch or sugar.
- **Your success:** Jot down your weight and, more important, any new behavior. Have you started eating breakfast consistently? Did you add more steps to your daily walking? Did you make over your snacks? Are you feeling less hungry in the evening? Write down these important milestones in your notebook so you can review them whenever you're feeling unmotivated.

I'm guessing you've heard all of this before, and you're still not writing anything down. Let's shoot for a middle ground. You don't have to keep a weight-loss diary for the rest of your life. Promise yourself this much. You will:

1. Write in your diary every day for the first month.
2. Write in your diary the first week of every month afterward.

3. Return to journaling every day if your weight loss stalls or you begin to regain.

**3. Learn how to relax.** As you lose weight, life will go on. You will encounter family pressure, work issues, and other sources of stress. You don't have to put off buying a house, accepting a promotion at work, or adopting a child just because you are trying to lose weight, but you do need to learn how to better deal with stress so that these big life events don't unravel your resolve.

I don't prescribe one specific way to relax, because many different methods work for many different people. I've listed a number of stress-reducing methods here. Try one or all of them, and incorporate the most useful into your life on a regular basis.

- **Walking:** Exercise releases tension and elevates levels of brain chemicals that help you relax. Find a beautiful location to walk and go there regularly, especially at the time of day when you are most likely to eat out of stress.
- **Reading:** If you can become engrossed in a novel, the comics, or a magazine, your reading will temporarily remove you from the stress of your life.
- **Self-indulgence:** A massage or pedicure allows you to experience caring and human touch, which can go a long way to lowering your stress response. Don't reward yourself with food. Reward yourself with pleasure.
- **Calling a friend:** Vent about what's going on in your life. Often by talking it out, you'll feel better.
- **Formal relaxation:** A relaxation technique called *progressive muscle relaxation* helps you isolate and relax away tension. Sit in a chair or lie on your back. Starting at your feet and moving up to your head, tense and then relax various muscle groups. Tense them up as you inhale, and release as you exhale.
- **Breathing:** Breathe deeply through your nose and then exhale forcefully through your mouth. As you exhale, visualize yourself letting go of pent-up stress. If you are really anxious, add another element to your breathing. As you inhale and exhale, say the word *calm* silently to yourself. You may also find it helpful to fix your eyes on a set point, such as the point midway

between your eyes (known as your "third eye") or at the tip of your nose.

- **Laughing.** Watch a funny movie or sitcom, or call a friend who can easily get you to laugh.
- **Take a relaxation class.** Consider any number of classes such as yoga, meditation, or breathing.

- - - - - - - - - - - - - - - - - - - - - - - - - - - - - - - - - - - - - - - - - -

### The Skinny on . . . Why Most People Regain What They Lose; The Cause of Yo-Yo Dieting Revealed

Many people manage to maintain their weight loss for a while. Then they start to feel confident. They go to a celebration or a birthday party. They have a piece of cake. They have a really big piece, because it's a good cake. The sugar and fat floods their bloodstream. Insulin spikes.

They wake the next day. They are fatigued and hungrier than they've been for a very long time. They don't feel like making the omelet they usually have for breakfast. They get in the car and drive to a coffee shop and get a doughnut instead. More rapidly digested sugar comes in. Insulin spikes again. Hunger increases even more, and they think, "Uh-oh, here it comes again." They weigh themselves, and they think, "I'm up five pounds! How could I gain five pounds in one day and be so hungry? It's not worth it." They give up.

That's what causes "yo-yo" dieting. It's part physical (high levels of insulin) and part mental (demoralization). You can't fight the physical part unless you get back on the diet, or temporarily take a medicine, but you can fight the mental part. The trick here is knowing that you can't gain 5 pounds in one day. It's impossible. What you've gained is water, and maybe a half pound of fat, at most. If you get back on the plan, your eating and weight will get under control, slowly and surely. It may take a week, but you will get back there, so don't give up. In chapter 11, I've included precise advice to help you get back on track when you wake up the morning after eating cake or another insulin-spiking food. You can stop the weight-loss, weight-regain cycle. I'll show you how.

**4. Create a reward system.** My patients are often their harshest critics. They say things like "I was wrong to do that" and "I let myself down." I hope by now you know that this isn't your fault. You are battling a disease, and the battle is going to be an intense one. You will slip up from time to time. That's why I want you to create a reward system, but not a system that rewards you for pounds lost on the scale. Focus on what's in your control: your behavior. You can control what you eat, but you can't control how much you weigh. If you never eat breakfast, and you manage to eat breakfast twice in your first week of the plan, that's cause for celebration, not self-flagellation! Reward yourself for consistently making each of the dietary and lifestyle changes in Part 2 of this book. Choose a motivating reward that does not center on food. Perhaps you buy a new outfit, get a pedicure, or take a long weekend.

## How to Eat for Fullness

*The Skinny's* initial eating plan is strict. It includes no rapidly digested starch (you'll have one portion of a whole-grain, high-fiber, slow-digesting starch with dinner) or sugar, and a minimum of dietary fat. The low amount of rapidly digested starch will help drive down insulin and leptin levels, allowing your brain and muscle cells to regain their full level of function and overcome fullness resistance. The hearty amounts of protein and fiber will reduce levels of the hunger hormone ghrelin, filling you up on fewer calories.

The eating plan is designed to allow you to eat a high volume of food, but consume a low number of calories. Your breakfast, lunch, and dinner plate will not resemble those tiny portions you see at *nouveau cuisine* restaurants. Rather, you'll consume four to eight egg whites in your omelets for breakfast and three-course lunches and dinners. You can follow up with one or two snacks a day, too, as needed. You won't be eating less. If anything, you'll be eating more.

Before I list the food choices for breakfast, lunch, dinner, and snacks, I'd like to go over a few do's and don'ts.

**Do:** Eat the full amount of food suggested for breakfast. Many people make the mistake of eating too little for breakfast, sometimes in a misguided attempt to cut calories and speed weight loss. This only backfires later in the day when their hunger and cravings peak, causing them to dive into the cookies and other high-calorie treats.

**Do:** Eat out. You don't have to cook all of your meals at home in order to lose weight. You'll find detailed eating-out suggestions in chapters 5 and 7.

**Do:** Eat as many vegetables as you can. These are free foods. If you are hungry between meals or at the end of a meal, have celery, zucchini, carrots, peppers, cauliflower, or broccoli (see the list of recommended vegetables in chapter 13). Eat them cooked or raw. Dip them in salsa for added zip. Many of my patients like to eat a large mound of sautéed bean sprouts whenever they feel hungry or unsatisfied. They tell me that the texture reminds them of rice, but at only 30 calories per 8 ounces, the sprouts are much more filling for a fraction of the calories.

**Do:** Flavor your meals with fresh or dried herbs and spices, salsa, vinegar, and mustard. These are unlimited. You need not measure them. Use the low-calorie dressing and sauce recipes in chapter 12, too. You can also use pickles, but they are high in sodium, so avoid them if you are on a salt-restricted diet.

**Do:** Try to drink water, unsweetened tea or green tea, or plain or flavored seltzer before each meal. It helps fill you up. You don't need to drink a specific amount each day.

**Do:** Continue to consume a modest amount of caffeine. Coffee and tea contain no calories, and the caffeine may reduce appetite and speed your metabolism. It perplexes me why some diets require people to give up caffeine, especially considering that the withdrawal produces irritability, restlessness, muscle stiffness, poor concentration, headaches, and even chills. Those are not symptoms you want to battle as you are concentrating on making dietary changes. I do recommend, however, that you cap your caffeine consumption at three servings a day. Consuming more than that amount may disturb sleep and make you feel anxious.

**Do:** Continue to drink alcohol, but try to hold yourself to one drink a day. That's 12 ounces of beer, 5 ounces of wine, or 1½ ounces of spirits. Alcohol has an appetizing effect that can cause you to eat more if you drink on an empty stomach. Have your drink with your main course and not before your meal because it can make you hungrier.

**Do:** Eat from appetizer-size plates. Research shows that small plates make food seem larger, and our eyes are just as much involved in appetite as our stomachs. If your eyes think you are eating a lot, so does your brain.

**Do:** Eat slowly. Slower eating allows fullness signals more time to reach your brain. Try to put down your flatware between bites, chew food thoroughly, and notice the taste and texture of your food.

**Don't:** Torture yourself. Just because I do not include sugar and include very little starch on the Phase 1 plan does not mean you must continually feel deprived. As soon as you tell yourself that you can "never" eat a certain food, a strange thing happens. You crave it all the more. Don't build a shrine to any food. If you want a dessert or a starch, have it, but follow this advice:

- Choose the healthiest, highest-fiber option. I'm talking about whole-grain bread, wild or brown rice, quinoa, and small new potatoes with the skin. Research shows that these types of high-fiber starchy foods do not tend to cause the rebound hunger that their refined, quickly digesting cousins do. In fact, Swedish researchers determined that consuming a high-fiber starch with dinner resulted in improved metabolism and reduced appetite the following day. In particular, a hormone called adiponectin was higher the morning after participants consumed high-fiber starch (barley-kernel bread) than when they consumed rapidly digested starch (white bread). This hormone improves insulin sensitivity and prevents heart disease.
- If possible, choose desserts with a little nutrition, such as an oatmeal raisin cookie or dark chocolate with a high cacao content.
- Measure out your starch or dessert before eating. Your portions should be no larger than the following: ½ cup whole-grain starch (barley, brown rice, wild rice, whole-grain pasta), one slice of whole-grain bread, two slices of light or low-carb whole-grain bread, half of a whole-wheat pita, one mini whole-wheat pita, one multigrain English muffin, three small new potatoes. Consult the list of recommended desserts and their portion sizes in chapter 13. If consuming a large ice cream dessert, share it with your dinner partner.
- Always eat starch and dessert after you've consumed protein, and ideally at the end of dinner. In other words, eat filling foods first and fattening foods last. When you have fattening foods after eating your vegetables and protein, they have less effect on your appetite. That's the key to long-term success.
- Make sugar an occasional or a weekly indulgence rather than a daily indulgence.

### The Skinny on . . . Why Cheat Meals Backfire

Some diets suggest that you follow their eating recommendations flawlessly until the weekend, eat whatever you want all weekend long, and then get back on track on Monday. Others give you a cheat night, and still others a daily cheat meal. These approaches just don't work because they encourage you to build a shrine to a particular food or food group. As you wait out your craving until it's time to cheat, that food grows more and more palpable in your mind. Then, when you do dig in, you eat a much larger portion than usual. Worse, the huge intake of sugar and/or starch triggers rebound hunger, so you continue to overeat. You wake the next morning with a food coma. You're tired, starving, and craving sweets, and instead of having a nutritious breakfast, you cheat more by having a doughnut. It's much better to have sugar or starch in controlled amounts, if you feel the urge, but only after you've consumed vegetables and protein.

**Don't:** Cheat at breakfast. This is the most important meal to do right because it will affect your hunger for the rest of the day. Breakfast is the most potent appetite suppressant you can give yourself.

## The Phase 1 Plan (Duration: 3+ Months)

Use the following menus to guide your eating for Phase 1. Follow this plan for at least three months. Use these guidelines to decide when to move on to Phase 2:

- If you lose more than 1 percent of your body weight per week, switch to Phase 2 menus, even if you've been following Phase 1 for fewer than three months. This speed of weight loss is too rapid to maintain.
- If, after three months, you still have a significant amount of weight to lose and you do not feel deprived or bored, you may continue with Phase 1 even longer. If you feel deprived

or have intense cravings for starch, however, move on to Phase 2.

- If your weight plateaus and you decide to maintain rather than try to lose more, transition to Phase 2. On the other hand, if your weight plateaus long before your three months is up, and you still have much more weight to lose, stay in Phase 1 and read chapter 10 to see if you have a hidden barrier to weight loss.

Note that some people do fine on Phase 1, but develop cravings when they progress to Phase 2! As soon as they reintroduce too much starch or sugar, they develop cravings to eat even more. If this happens to you, shift your eating back to Phase 1. Phase 1 may be strict, but as long as you are eating plenty of vegetables and healthy proteins, it's perfectly healthy and you can follow it for the rest of your life if needed.

## Phase 1 Breakfast Options

Keep breakfast high in protein and low in starch. Give yourself bonus points for consuming a few veggies with breakfast, but don't drive yourself crazy slicing and dicing in the early morning hours. The most important nutrient for your first meal is protein. You'll consume plenty of wholesome vegetables at lunch and dinner.

You may add an unlimited amount of vegetables to any option. Choose one:

---

Vegetable omelet: 4 to 8 egg whites (or ½ cup to 1 cup egg substitute) mixed with chopped vegetables of your choice in any quantity

---

Cheese omelet: 4 to 8 egg whites (or ½ cup to 1 cup egg substitute) with 1 slice low-fat cheese

---

Lean protein omelet: 4 to 8 egg whites (or ½ cup to 1 cup egg substitute) with 1 ounce lean ham, roast beef, turkey breast, chicken breast, crabmeat, or another lean protein source

---

Asparagus Omelet (page 170)

---

Egg-White Frittata (page 171)

---

Morning Shake (page 171)

---

1 cup 1% cottage cheese mixed with 1 cup strawberries, 1 cup cubed melon, ⅓ cup blueberries, or 1 sliced medium peach and 1 tablespoon ground flax or dry-roasted or raw pumpkin or sunflower seeds

6 to 8 ounces nonfat Greek yogurt (such as Fage brand) with 1 cup strawberries or ¾ cup blueberries, blackberries, or raspberries

3 turkey sausage links with ½ grapefruit

2 to 3 slices lean ham or turkey rolled with 1 slice cheese

4 hard-boiled egg whites with 15 almonds or cashews or 25 peanuts or pistachios

4 hard-boiled egg whites with 1 cup watermelon, honeydew, or cantaloupe

A commercially prepared protein shake. Look for shakes that contain 150 to 210 calories and 12 to 25 grams of protein. They should contain fewer than 9 grams of fat, 25 grams of carbohydrate, and 18 grams of sugar. Atkins Advantage and Slim-Fast Low-Carb Meals shakes meet these criteria.

1 apple with 2 low-fat string cheeses

1 apple with 2 tablespoons crunchy nut butter

1 to 2 scoops Carnation Instant Breakfast Carb Conscious, Designer Protein, or Genisoy protein powder mixed with 8 ounces skim milk

3 ounces smoked salmon (lox) and 1 to 2 Laughing Cow Light Cheese wedges

## Phase 1 Lunch Options

Ideally, consume lunch in the order specified: appetizer, side dish, and then main course, but don't drive yourself crazy. It's perfectly acceptable to choose one-dish meals such as grilled chicken salads or tuna over a bed of lettuce. You'll find eating-out options in chapter 5.

| Appetizer | Salad made with unlimited greens and chopped vegetables (at least 1 cup), with 1 tablespoon olive oil and vinegar, 1 tablespoon regular vinaigrette, 2 tablespoons fat-free dressing, or 1 serving of any salad dressing recipe in chapter 12 |
| --- | --- |
| Vegetable side dish | Unlimited raw, steamed, roasted, or lightly sautéed vegetables (at least 1 cup). Consult the list of recommended vegetables (page 203) and the vegetable side dish recipes in chapter 12. |

| Main course | Any main-course recipe in chapter 12 or 5 to 8 ounces of lean protein, more if you're still hungry. Good lean protein options include the following:<br><br>• Skinless chicken breast<br>• Turkey breast<br>• Water-packed tuna<br>• Any fish, shellfish, or sardines<br>• Soy or turkey burger (no roll) |
|---|---|

## Phase 1 Snack Options

Consume one to two snacks a day, as needed. You may accompany any snack with an unlimited amount of vegetables. Recommended snacks include the following:

1 cup fresh berries or melon cubes

½ grapefruit

1 whole apple, nectarine, or plum

6 to 12 almonds or cashews, 10 to 20 small peanuts, or 4 to 8 walnut halves

4 ounces 1% cottage cheese

8 ounces low-fat plain or artificially sweetened yogurt (90 to 120 calories per container)

½ cup fat-free, sugar-free pudding (made from the mix, not the premade snack cup)

⅔ cup edamame

Unlimited amount of raw vegetables

2 wedges Laughing Cow Light Cheese on 2 celery sticks

1 cup carrot or celery sticks with 2 tablespoons hummus

1 sliced apple with 2 teaspoons peanut butter

1 pear and 5 whole cashews

1 ounce part-skim mozzarella cheese and 4 Triscuits

½ cup 1% cottage cheese with cinnamon and 4 walnut halves

1 ounce reduced-fat cheddar cheese with 1 cup fresh berries

½ cup 1% cottage cheese topped with 1 sliced kiwi and cinnamon

8 ounces artificially sweetened yogurt and 1½ tablespoons trail mix

12 ounces nonfat café latte sprinkled with cinnamon and 6 almonds on the side

1 Ryvita or Wasa cracker with 1 cup canned ready-to-serve bean soup, Lentil Soup (page 184), Easiest Vegetable Soup (page 183), Gazpacho (page 184), or Tuscan White Bean Soup (page 188)

1 cup salad greens with ¼ cup each chickpeas and kidney beans, with 1 tablespoon vinaigrette

## Phase 1 Dinner Options

Ideally, consume dinner in the order specified: appetizer, side dish, and then main course. It's perfectly acceptable to consume one-dish meals such as chicken stir-fry, a big salad, or a casserole that does not contain starch. You'll find eating-out options in chapter 7.

| | |
|---|---|
| Appetizers (choose up to three) | • Clear broth<br>• Miso soup<br>• Easiest Vegetable Soup (page 183) or canned vegetable soup<br>• Gazpacho (page 184)<br>• Lentil Soup (page 184)<br>• Salad made with unlimited greens and chopped vegetables, with 1 teaspoon olive oil and vinegar, 1 tablespoon regular vinaigrette, 2 tablespoons fat-free dressing, or 1 serving of any salad dressing recipe in chapter 12<br>• Shrimp or seafood cocktail |
| Vegetable side dish | Consult the list of recommended vegetables in chapter 13 and the vegetable side-dish recipes in chapter 12. Consume at least 1 cup. |
| Main course | Any main-course recipe in chapter 12 or 5 to 8 ounces of lean protein, more if you're still hungry. Good lean protein options include the following:<br><br>• Skinless chicken breast<br>• Turkey breast<br>• Water-packed tuna<br>• Any fish, shellfish, or sardines<br>• Soy or turkey burger (no roll)<br>• Lean beef (London broil, filet mignon, flank steak)*<br>• Veal*<br>• Lamb*<br>• Pork tenderloin*<br>• Fresh baked ham*<br>*No more than two to three times a week |

| Starch side dish | Choose one: |
| --- | --- |
| | • ½ cup barley, buckwheat, bulgur wheat, or quinoa<br>• ½ cup long-grain brown or wild rice<br>• ½ cup whole-wheat pasta or soba noodles<br>• ½ cup lentils or beans |

## The Phase 2 Plan (Duration: The Rest of Your Life)

Move on to Phase 2 once you reach a plateau, have reached your goal weight, or feel bored with the Phase 1 options. Phase 2 is how you should eat on most days on an ongoing basis. It will become your maintenance diet. As you transition to Phase 2 eating, you'll add one daily serving of starch a week for three weeks.

When increasing starch, choose high-fiber options. These options usually have the word *whole* on the packaging, such as whole-grain bread, whole-grain couscous, whole-grain bulgur, and whole-grain pasta. Most important, look at the number of grams of fiber per serving. If it's 0, that's not what I would call whole-grain. Look for 3 or more grams of fiber per 80-calorie serving. In addition to fiber, these whole foods contain important plant nutrients such as lignans, phenolic acids, phytoestrogens, and antioxidants that reduce your risk for heart disease, diabetes, cancer, and stroke.

Also pay attention to how the grains are processed. Steel-cut oatmeal, small nuggets with the bran intact, has a far lower glycemic load than instant rolled oats, which have a high glycemic load.

Everyone's body is different. Some people can add just one starch serving, others two, and still

**Skinny Mini:** Don't be fooled by food marketers. If you see the word *multigrain* on the packaging, it doesn't necessarily mean the product is whole grain or high in fiber. Some multigrain products, especially bread, simply contain a mixture of three or more refined grains. Rye and pumpernickel bread are not necessarily whole grain either. Look for the word *whole* in front of those grains, too. Quinoa and oatmeal are always whole grain. The word *whole* will not appear on packaging for these products.

others three. You may be able to occasionally get away with more starch—such as four daily servings—but these days must stay in the occasional category. If you try to consume four starch servings a day, you may regain.

As you add starch servings, carefully monitor your weight, your appetite, and your cravings for sweets. Weigh yourself every day. Also, keep a detailed food log, writing down what you eat and your hunger levels before, after, and between meals. If you find yourself feeling hungrier after increasing your starch servings, you need to back off. The same goes for weight gain. Think of each change you make as an experiment. If you want to eat cold cereal every day, then try it. Make an experiment out of it, but notice how hungry you feel. If you start feeling excessively hungry, use that feedback to modify what you eat.

Follow these do's and don'ts for Phase 2 eating:

**Do:** Transition to Phase 2 in steps. Add one starch serving at lunch, after you've finished the rest of the meal. This is the best time to reintroduce starch because you will already feel somewhat full from your vegetables and protein.

Wait a week and notice how you feel. Then add a starch serving at a snack. Then, occasionally, include starch with breakfast.

**Do:** Eat starch last. At dinner, have starch only after your appetizer, vegetables, and main course. At lunch, eat bread last, after you've consumed everything else.

**Don't:** Eat starch if you are not hungry. If the rest of the meal fills you up, don't eat it just because it's there.

**Don't:** Add starch for every meal at once. Do it one meal at a time.

**Don't:** Consistently include starch with breakfast. The occasional slice of whole-grain toast with your breakfast meal may be okay, but try to keep breakfast a strict combination of lean protein with optional vegetables.


## Phase 2 Breakfast Options

Ideally, you should choose Phase 1 options most of the time. In a pinch, the following options are high enough in fiber that they should still control hunger most of the morning. Pay careful attention to how you feel after introducing these options. Also carefully measure cold cereal. Many people pour more than ½ cup into a bowl, and overeating cereal may leave you feeling hungry rather than full. If you begin to feel hungrier after introducing these breakfasts, go back to the original Phase 1 choices. Remember, you don't have to have these daily, just occasionally.

Choose one:

---

½ cup high-fiber cereal (see chapter 13 for recommended brands) with ¾ cup skim milk

---

Slow-cooking oatmeal (such as McCann's Irish Oatmeal brand) with up to ¾ cup skim milk and 1 sliced peach or ⅓ cup berries

---

Egg sandwich: 1 whole-wheat English muffin with 4 to 6 egg whites

---

1 whole-wheat English muffin with 1½ tablespoons crunchy peanut butter or other nut butter

---

## Phase 2 Lunch Options

You may consume all of the Phase 1 options plus the following side dishes.

- 1 slice whole-grain bread (at least 3 grams of fiber per slice; the more the better)
- 2 slices light whole-grain bread (at least 1.5 grams of fiber per slice)
- 1 slice rye or pumpernickel bread
- Half of a whole-wheat pita
- 1 mini whole-wheat pita
- 1 multigrain light English muffin (at least 8 grams of fiber per muffin)

## Phase 2 Snack Options

You may consume all of the Phase 1 snack options, plus the following. Consume these snacks later in the afternoon or after dinner, not in the morning. You may pair these options with an unlimited amount of vegetables.

- 3 cups microwave light popcorn
- 2 slices Ryvita or Wasa cracker
- 5 whole-wheat Triscuits
- 3 Graham cracker squares with 2 teaspoons peanut butter

# What to Expect

Going from cheese doodles and hot dogs to salads and chicken breast will make you feel different. Your body has grown accustomed to your eating habits, your lifestyle habits, and your weight. As a result, when you try to change these habits, you may experience withdrawal symptoms, particularly as you wean yourself off sugar, because it's addictive.

Starch may also be addictive. I had a patient who went to a hypnotist to help himself stop smoking and eating sugar. He stopped eating sugar, but he started gaining weight, and that's when he came to see me. Yes, he'd stopped the sweets, but he'd replaced them with bread, pasta, potatoes, and other starchy carbs. He was eating larger portions of starch than he was of sweets, and he was gaining as a result.

For these reasons, expect the initial three to five days of this dietary change to be a little rougher than usual. You may get headaches, feel fatigued, or not quite be yourself. These symptoms are temporary, and they lift for most people. Minimize them by tackling the plan in a step-by-step approach. The small incremental changes I suggest will slowly wean you off sugar and starch, replacing those addictions with fiber-, protein-, and nutrient-dense foods. This slow transition will keep most withdrawal symptoms to a minimum.

Which brings me to my next point. This plan will definitely reduce many of the barriers that have prevented you from being successful in the past, but it's not magic. I know about those diets that promise that you can lose all the weight you want or lose it in record time. You know what I say? If all these claims were really true, everyone in the world would fit into a size six. You've probably bought into such exaggerated claims more times than you'd care to admit. It's normal to want fast, dramatic results. The weight-loss industry has trained you to buy into such promises. I'm an honest person, though, so I'm not going to promise you anything that I can't back up.

With this plan, many people are able to lose between 10 and 20 percent of their weight, and most can lose 7 percent or more. With my approach, you may not lose startling amounts of weight within a week or even within a month. The weight will come off slowly, because you will implement changes slowly in order to get the weight off.

Here's more. This plan allows you to know what it feels like to fill up on a normal amount of food. You will eventually be able to stop obsessing about food. You will eventually feel full on cue, so you can put down

## The Skinny on . . . Why Weight Loss Slows over Time

You may lose 10 pounds during the first week on this or any other plan, but that's nothing to celebrate. Most of the initial dramatic loss on any diet stems from lost water and muscle, not from fat. The pounds that the average dieter loses during the first few days of a diet are composed of 70 percent water, 5 percent muscle protein, and 25 percent fat. Gradually, over time, the amount of lost water and protein goes down, and the amount of fat goes up. After about a month of dieting, the average person is losing 25 percent protein and water and 75 percent fat. Fat is calorie dense, and besides making hormones, its major role is to store calories for later use. One pound of fat contains more than 4,000 calories, whereas a pound of muscle stores only about 1,800. If you're burning more fat, your rate of weight loss will slow because you need to burn more calories to lose a pound.

your fork before you overeat. You'll be able to stop forcing yourself to eat less because you'll eat less automatically. Think about how freeing that will feel. Think about how much more mental energy you'll have when you won't have to talk yourself through each meal. Then think about turning the page and getting started.

# Part Two

## Skinny Makeovers

# 4

# The Skinny Breakfast Makeover

Helene was back in my office roughly nine months after she'd lost weight. "I'm gaining back the weight and I don't know why," she told me.

"How are you eating?" I asked.

"I'm hardly eating anything," she said. With some more questioning, I learned that Helene was indeed eating very little before 6 P.M. Her life had gotten busy, and she'd slipped back into an old bad habit of having only coffee for breakfast and a very small lunch. Every evening she promised to stay away from the chips and sweets, but her nightly scenario was the same. As she prepared dinner, her control unraveled. She'd start nibbling as she put the meal together and she usually didn't stop eating until bedtime.

I listened as she questioned her resolve. "I don't know why I continually lose my willpower at night," she said. "I can't seem to stay in control."

"I'd like you to make just one change. I think it's going to help you a lot," I said. "I'd like you to start eating breakfast again."

She looked at me thoughtfully. "That's right. I stopped eating breakfast," she said. "That's why I'm so hungry at night."

Then she paused.

"But I'm not hungry in the morning. I don't think I can eat. Shouldn't I first try to rein in my eating at night?"

"How long have you been trying to eat less at night?" I asked.

"A month," she said.

"Is it working?"

"I guess not," she said.

To ease her into the breakfast habit, I suggested she drink a meal replacement beverage rather than cook a hot meal. "You don't have to drink the whole thing at once," I said. "You can sip it over the course of the morning."

She took my advice, and within just a few days she felt better. She was in control at night and hungry in the morning.

## Why It Works

If you find the motivation to make only one dietary change, this is the one to make. Consider the following:

- Seventy-eight percent of people who successfully lose weight and keep it off eat breakfast every day, according to the National Weight Control Registry, a database of more than 5,000 people who have lost more than 30 pounds and kept it off for at least a year.
- Of thousands of participants in an English study, those who consumed the most calories at breakfast weighed less than those who didn't eat breakfast or who ate very little for this morning meal.
- Breakfast eaters in a Harvard study were less likely to gain weight over ten years than non–breakfast eaters.

You may think that skipping this one daily meal will help you eat fewer calories, but it rarely works out that way. Instead, skipping breakfast merely shifts your caloric intake to later in the day. What should be lunch becomes your breakfast. What should be dinner becomes your lunch. What should be hours of not eating before bedtime becomes a snacking gorge. People who skip breakfast tend to consume more than half of their daily calories at night. For example, I recently counseled a patient who told me, "I don't know why I'm gaining weight. I eat nothing." He skipped breakfast, had a small salad for lunch, and ate very small portions at dinner. But he kept a package of Good & Plenty on his bedside table. Whenever he woke in the middle of the night, he'd snack from the bag. He finished a 5-pound bag every two weeks, consuming hundreds of calories of candy each night.

This type of late-night eating, recent research finds, nudges triglycerides up during sleep, contributing to fat storage and fullness resistance.

Omitting breakfast may contribute to insulin resistance, too. When women skipped breakfast in a University of Nottingham study, their insulin levels were higher and the hormone was less effective than when they ate breakfast. LDL ("bad") cholesterol also rose. Again, insulin resistance leads to leptin resistance and therefore fullness resistance.

**Skinny Solution:** If you overdo it at night—say by having a huge dessert—you'll wake the following morning with a food hangover. You'll feel tired. You may have a headache, and you'll be hungrier than usual. It's extremely important, on such mornings, to eat a breakfast that strictly adheres to the Phase 1 menu options. This meal will help normalize fullness hormone levels, so you're less likely to follow a night of overindulgence with a day of overeating. You'll find more advice for getting back on track after overindulging in chapter 11.

When you eat breakfast daily, on the other hand, you control appetite and cravings. You improve insulin sensitivity, turning down your appetite all day long. You'll automatically eat less for lunch, snacks, and dinner. The right type of breakfast can even speed up your metabolic rate, so you burn more calories throughout the day.

## How to Do It

Research shows that eating fast-digesting, starchy, or sweet carbohydrates such as muffins, bagels, or juice can increase your appetite later in the day. On the other hand, many studies link protein consumption—particularly when eaten as part of the day's first meal—with a reduced appetite throughout the day. Eating protein-rich foods for breakfast will help you more easily make better choices for snacks, lunch, and dinner.

Just in case you're not willing to take my word for it (and I'm not offended), I'd like to tell you about some research that backs up what I'm suggesting. In one study, completed at Saint Louis University, thirty overweight women ate the same number of calories at breakfast, either from eggs (which are high in protein) or from bagels (which are high in carbohydrate). During the 3½ hours between breakfast and lunch, the women who ate eggs felt more satisfied and less hungry than the women who ate bagels. Without trying, they ate roughly 140 fewer calories at lunch than the bagel eaters, and continued to eat less food for the following 36 hours! Studies show that this protein-induced reduction in appetite occurs no matter your age, sex, or weight.

Make your breakfast either 100 percent protein or a combination of protein and high-fiber carbohydrate foods. You don't, however, have to put a huge emphasis on eating fiber-rich foods for breakfast. Both protein and fiber are important, but protein is the most important nutrient to consume in the morning. If you don't have a lot of time in the morning, don't worry about chopping vegetables for an omelet. Have a protein shake.

Let's talk about the specific benefits of some of the foods you'll find featured on the plan.

**Eggs:** One egg provides 7 grams of protein. The whites are the most concentrated form of protein available. I recommend whites because they allow you to consume a greater volume of food for a smaller amount of calories with less unhealthy saturated fat and cholesterol. Some of my patients turn up their noses at egg-white omelets and scrambled egg whites. If this is the case, you may mix one whole egg into your egg whites. You won't be able to tell the difference.

Use this advice to make better-tasting egg-white meals:

* Add flavor with low-fat cheese or lean ham. You can mix egg whites with almost any food you love, including lean turkey or chicken, smoked salmon, crabmeat, shrimp, shredded low-fat cheese, peppers, mushrooms, tomatoes, asparagus . . . the list goes on and on. See the recipes in chapter 12 for cooking ideas.

- Whisk a teaspoon or more (to taste) of your favorite spice blend into the eggs before cooking. This better distributes the flavor than sprinkling it on top just before serving.
- Usually I recommend that you cook with cooking spray. This reduces the amount of oil and calories. Egg whites cook quickly and often stick to the pan, so in this one instance, I suggest you use ½ teaspoon oil. The oil will also add a little flavor to the eggs and prevent the bottom side of your omelet from becoming overly crispy.
- For fluffier omelets, beat eggs at room temperature and stir in a tablespoon of skim milk or water into the whites as you beat them.

**Protein shakes:** I generally consider real food—such as eggs and cottage cheese—to be better for your health than processed foods. Real foods contain wholesome nutrients that no processed food can emulate. That said, a protein shake made from whey or soy protein is definitely healthier than eating fast food or breakfast pastries.

Use the Morning Shake recipe (page 171) or keep a stash of commercially prepared protein shakes at home and at the office. You can grab these easy options on your way out the door and consume them during your commute. Because the shakes contain only about 180 calories, drink one for breakfast and another for a midmorning snack two to three hours later. My patients report that these shakes give them about two hours or more of staying power. Once you get hungry, it's time for another one.

If you have trouble stomaching protein shakes, check the label. Study participants at North Carolina State University preferred the taste and texture of high-protein meal-replacement beverages that contained whey protein or a combination of soy and whey protein over shakes that contained soy protein alone.

Do you wonder, "What happens when I stop using the shakes?" Perhaps you're thinking, "Oprah regained all the weight she lost with Optifast. Won't I gain back the weight, too?" Not necessarily.

First, I'm not suggesting you drink five shakes a day and eat no solid food like those 800-calorie liquid diets of yesteryear. In this case, you're using the shake only as a breakfast meal replacement, almost like a liquid appetite suppressant. The shake isn't something you use to lose weight and then stop drinking once you start maintaining. It's a breakfast option, just as eggs are a breakfast option. I don't think there's any reason to stop using them as part of your regular plan, even after you've reached maintenance. You can continue to use breakfast shakes for the rest of your life and stay healthy. As long as you're eating real food—vegetables and healthy protein—at your other meals, you have nothing to worry about.

**Skinny Solution:** Some people find that they do better if they consume hot food for lunch and a shake with cooked vegetables for dinner. They feel more in control at night if they stick to a shake rather than sit down to a hot meal.

Second, the eating approaches in this book work only if you follow them. If you're too busy to prepare meals, then you need another option, and meal-replacement beverages provide that option. Many of these beverages are cheaper than eating real food. They're also healthier than you may think, especially if they replace unhealthy conveniences such as fast food, doughnuts, and toaster pastries. They are so convenient, you don't even have to put them in the toaster.

Most important: they work. Many of my patients tell me that these beverages are like appetite suppressants in a can. They feel hungry, drink one, and immediately feel full. After consuming one, they can control cravings for the fattening foods they usually eat.

You may replace up to two meals a day with a commercially prepared shake. Because each one contains only about 160 calories, it will fill you up for only three to four hours. Once you feel hungry again, have another shake as a between-meals snack. Consume up to three shakes a day. A typical shake-drinking schedule may look like this:

| | |
|---|---|
| 9:30 A.M. | Shake |
| Noon | Cooked vegetables or salad plus shake (if needed) |
| 2:00 P.M. | Shake |
| 5:00 P.M. | Shake |
| 7:30 P.M. | Dinner: 5 to 8 ounces of protein with a plate of vegetables and/or salad |
| Midevening | Snack (vegetables) |

Don't try to speed weight loss by consuming just shakes and no solid food. Solid food contains important nutrients that just can't be put in even the most brilliantly designed beverages or bars, because we don't know what all of them are. You also want to stay in the habit of eating solid foods. If you consume liquid meals for months on end, solid food will taste incredibly delicious once you start eating again. Keeping at least one solid meal in your daily repertoire prevents you from feeling deprived and from going hog wild when you eat solid foods.

**Cottage Cheese:** It's rich in protein, with low-fat versions supplying 16 grams for every 100 calories. Choose low-fat versions, as the higher-fat varieties supply an overabundance of calories. One cup of whole-milk cottage cheese, for instance, provides 216 calories, whereas low-fat cottage cheese made with 1% milk has only 163. Yet both provide the same volume of food. You'll feel just as satisfied after eating the low-fat version, at a savings of more than 40 calories.

I recommend the following options during Phase 1. Please keep in mind that most people eat too little at breakfast rather than too much. If you feel hungry midmorning after switching over to these *Skinny* breakfast options, you're probably not eating enough. Do one of the following:

- Add more egg whites to your omelets or mix more vegetables into them.
- Make sure you are eating the full serving suggested.
- Have a shake with one of the other choices.

Skinny Mini: On three separate occasions, Swiss researchers fed fifteen men one of three meals: a high-carbohydrate meal, a balanced carbohydrate and protein meal, and a high-protein meal. Then they gave the men a series of brainteasers to complete throughout the morning to test their memory. (Think of the game, "I'm going on a picnic and I'm bringing apples, bananas, and cantaloupe," and you have a rough idea of what the researchers put these guys through.) The men did best on these tests after eating the high-protein and balanced meals and worst after the high-carbohydrate meal, possibly because the carbohydrate meal caused blood sugar levels to rise and then crash.

You may accompany any option with an unlimited amount of vegetables. Choose one:

---

Vegetable omelet: 4 to 8 egg whites (or ½ cup to 1 cup egg substitute) mixed with chopped vegetables of your choice in any quantity

---

Cheese omelet: 4 to 8 egg whites (or ½ cup to 1 cup egg substitute) with 1 slice low-fat cheese

---

Lean protein omelet: 4 to 8 egg whites (or ½ cup to 1 cup egg substitute) with 1 ounce lean ham, roast beef, turkey breast, chicken breast, crabmeat, or another lean protein source

---

Asparagus Omelet (page 170)

---

Egg-White Frittata (page 171)

---

Morning Shake (page 171)

---

1 cup 1% cottage cheese mixed with 1 cup strawberries, 1 cup cubed melon, ⅓ cup blueberries, or 1 sliced medium peach and 1 tablespoon ground flax or dry-roasted or raw pumpkin or sunflower seeds

---

6 to 8 ounces nonfat Greek yogurt (such as Fage brand) with 1 cup strawberries or ¾ cup blueberries, blackberries, or raspberries

---

3 turkey sausage links with ½ grapefruit

---

2 to 3 slices lean ham or turkey rolled with 1 slice cheese

---

4 hard-boiled egg whites with 15 almonds or cashews or 25 peanuts or pistachios

---

4 hard-boiled egg whites with 1 cup watermelon, honeydew, or cantaloupe

---

A commercially prepared protein shake. Look for shakes that contain 150 to 210 calories and 12 to 25 grams of protein. They should contain fewer than 9 grams of fat, 25 grams of carbohydrate, and 18 grams of sugar. Atkins Advantage and Slim-Fast Low-Carb Meals shakes meet these criteria.

---

1 apple with 2 low-fat string cheeses

---

1 apple with 2 tablespoons crunchy nut butter

---

1 to 2 scoops Carnation Instant Breakfast Carb Conscious, Designer Protein, or Genisoy protein powder mixed with 8 ounces skim milk

---

3 ounces smoked salmon (lox) and 1 to 2 Laughing Cow Light Cheese wedges

---

## What About Cereal and Oatmeal?

You may try oatmeal or high-fiber cold cereal in Phase 2. I don't recommend these options during Phase 1 because they may stimulate your appetite late in the day. Even during Phase 2, I recommend them only as occasional options rather than everyday meals. Have cereal or oats as often as once a week, but pay careful attention to how you feel. If you notice yourself feeling hungrier and craving sweets, then it's probably a better idea to stick with protein breakfast options.

If you consume cereal or oatmeal, use this advice:

**Measure the serving.** Most people can't measure with their eyes, so put a ⅓-cup measuring cup inside your cereal box and use it to dish out your cereal portion.

**Choose only cereals that are high in fiber.** Fiber is the appetite antidote for carbohydrate foods. Usually, starchy foods increase appetite, but if you pair starch with enough fiber, they don't. For example, high-fiber cereals slow stomach emptying and slow the absorption of sugar into the bloodstream, causing blood sugar and insulin to rise more evenly. The fiber also weighs down the stomach and intestines, instilling a sense of fullness.

Choose cereals with at least 5 grams of fiber (more is better; ideally more than 10), no more than 8 grams of added sugar, and no more than 200 calories per ½ cup. I recommend a number of cereal brands in chapter 13. Try the highest-fiber ones first, such as All-Bran and Fiber One. With 13 grams of fiber per ½ cup, these are the highest-fiber cereals on the market. My patients tell me that they feel stuffed after a ½-cup serving. If you don't like the taste of All-Bran, then try the Kashi options, which provide 8 to 10 grams of fiber per cup. Then try the Bran Flakes and other more moderate fiber options.

**Get slow-cooking oats.** Slow-cooking varieties such as McCann's Irish Oatmeal, steel-cut oats, or Quaker five-minute oats will satisfy you more than instant varieties. Instant oats have been stripped of most of their fiber; in essence, they are more like oat powder, so they digest more quickly. Steel-cut or Irish oatmeal, on the other hand, is made from whole, more coarse oats, so it contains more fiber and digests more slowly.

**Use only skim, skim plus, or 1% milk on your cereal.** Use skim plus if you feel you can't live without whole milk. I bet you can't tell the difference. Make sure to measure your milk. Most people measure liquids poorly with their eyes, and you want to use no more than

**Skinny Solution:** Going from no fiber to 12 grams can upset your stomach. If a high-fiber cereal upsets your stomach, cut back and increase gradually to 4 grams, then 8 grams, and even more as tolerated. You can do this by starting with lower-fiber options, or by mixing ½ cup high-fiber cereal with ¼ to ½ cup of your favorite brand. Pair this half-and-half cereal with lean protein, such as a hard-boiled egg (don't eat the yolk) or turkey sausage.

• • • • • • • • • • • • • • • • • • • • • • • • • • • • • • • • • • • • • • • •

¾ cup. The fat content in your milk can add many unnecessary calories to your breakfast, calories that do little to help you feel full. Consider these examples:

- ¾ cup heavy cream: 621 calories and 66.6 grams of fat (41 saturated)
- ¾ cup light cream: 351 calories and 34.7 grams of fat (21.6 saturated)
- ¾ cup half-and-half: 234 calories and 20.7 grams of fat (12.8 saturated)
- ¾ cup whole milk: 110 calories and 5.9 grams of fat (3.4 saturated)
- ¾ cup 2% milk: 97 calories and 3.6 grams of fat (2.3 saturated)
- ¾ cup 1% milk: 85 calories and 1.77 grams of fat (1.15 saturated)
- ¾ cup skim-plus milk: 82 calories and 0 grams of fat (0 saturated)
- ¾ cup skim milk: 67 calories and 0.1 gram of fat (0 saturated)

## What About Toast?

Again, I don't like to put any food in a "never" category. I'd prefer you kept breakfast to protein foods, but if you crave toast in the morning, let's make a compromise. Buy Thomas' Light Multi Grain English muffins. Each 100-calorie muffin contains 8 grams of fiber. Have one with a teaspoon or two of peanut butter.

If you use peanut butter, choose a full-fat, chunky variety. Despite popular belief, both regular and low-fat peanut butter contain the same number of calories, 94 per tablespoon. Reduced-fat peanut butter has less fat, but it has more sugar. The added sugar drives up blood sugar response after meals. Regular-fat versions have more fat but less sugar. They are more filling for the same amount of calories. Chunky versions are best because the small bits of whole peanuts take longer to digest than the puréed creamy versions, slowing digestion and reducing the glycemic response of your meal. Almond butter is another great option.

## What About Juice?

I don't recommend that my patients drink juice in the morning or any other time of day. Most juices are medium to high in glycemic load, dumping lots of sugar into your bloodstream at once, triggering rebound hunger. Our brains also don't easily respond to calories from liquids as they do to calories from solids. A 6-ounce glass of orange juice, for example, contains 75 calories, but few if any of those calories fill you up because liquids pass through your stomach too quickly to stimulate the stretch receptors that turn off appetite. A piece of fruit, on the other hand, contributes to fullness in a number of ways. It's heavy, so it weighs down your stomach. It contains fiber to slow the absorption of sugar into your bloodstream, and it requires chewing, which slows your eating pace. Ideally, choose fruit over fruit juice. If you really miss fruit

**Skinny Solution:** Many people spoon sugar onto cereal or oatmeal, which adds unnecessary calories that may trigger rebound hunger. Try cinnamon instead. Some of my patients consider it a nice alternative. A Pakistani study showed that people with type 2 diabetes who consumed a couple of tablespoons of cinnamon daily for 40 days had lower blood sugar, cholesterol, and triglyceride levels than people who didn't consume the spice.

juice, however, slowly wean yourself off by cutting your normal drink with water or seltzer. Have no more than 4 ounces, just enough to get the flavor.

## Make It Happen

It's one thing to tell you what to eat. It's another for you to put that advice into practice. I want you to succeed, which is why each of the chapters in Part 2 includes advice under the heading "Make It Happen." Consult the following excuses and solutions to them to help ease yourself into the breakfast habit.

### Excuse: I'm Too Busy

You'll make up for the small amount of time it takes to prepare and eat breakfast by being more productive throughout the day. People who consume low-GL breakfasts—such as the ones recommended in this plan—do better on tests of memory and attention than people who consume rapidly digested carbohydrates for breakfast. To make time for breakfast, use this advice:

**Wake up on time.** Set your alarm twenty to thirty minutes earlier so you can whip up a quick healthful meal.

**Plan a weekly breakfast menu.** The more you plan ahead, the more likely you'll find the time and energy to eat. Plan a week's worth of breakfast items before you go to the grocery store, then shop for all the ingredients while you are there so you have them on hand.

**Sit down.** Breakfast is one of those meals that people try to juggle with other tasks, such as driving, putting on makeup, or getting the kids ready for school. If you make breakfast relaxing and combine it with an activity you enjoy, such as reading the paper or watching TV, you'll more likely make time for it.

**Leave the preparation to someone else.** Put in a standing breakfast order at a local diner or restaurant and pick it up at the same time every morning on your way to work. Most restaurants offer egg whites or egg substitute, and you can even make fast food work. When no other option is available, consider getting an egg sandwich, but eat only the inside of the sandwich.

**Drink it.** Again, you need not make a complicated breakfast. If you're busy, stock up on protein shakes. Keep them at work, in your car, and on top of your fridge.

## Excuse: I'm Not Hungry

Ghrelin levels, in part, respond to habitual meal patterns. If you normally eat lunch at noon, for example, your ghrelin level will rise at noon. If you normally eat dinner at 7, it will rise at 7. If you start eating a midnight snack, for example, and continue to do so for a week or two, you'll start to feel hungry at midnight, even though your body definitely does not need calories at midnight.

Although this entrainment works against you with late-night snacking, it can work for you with breakfast. The first week or two of eating breakfast may feel challenging, but it will get easier over time as ghrelin entrains itself to this eating pattern. Eventually you'll wake up hungry.

You also may not feel hungry because you are eating too much at night. Habitual breakfast skippers tend to consume large dinners, followed by lots of late-night snacking. This late-night eating drives up triglyceride levels. These fats circulate in your bloodstream, and, because you are sleeping and not using your muscles, they tend to come to rest in your fat cells overnight. When you wake, you still feel full from your late-night snacks, skip breakfast again, and then set off another cycle.

Breaking this type of eating pattern will feel difficult in the beginning, but it will get easier over time. Start by consuming a small meal, such as a protein shake. If you can manage to drink only half of it at first, that's fine. Try to finish it over the course of the morning if you can. Gradually increase your consumption of the shake until you can consume the whole thing. By that time, your late-night snacking will probably have ebbed and you will be able to transition to solid breakfast foods.

# Fattening vs. Filling Foods

| Fattening Breakfast Options | Filling Breakfast Options | Why? |
|---|---|---|
| Refined bagel or bread with jelly | 100% whole-grain bread (one slice) with chunky peanut butter | The fiber in the whole-grain bread and the nuts in the peanut butter slow digestion, whereas the refined sugar in the jelly and the flour in the white bread drive up blood sugar and insulin, triggering rebound hunger. |
| Juice | 1 apple, peach, or pear; 1 cup berries; ½ grapefruit; 1 cup cubed melon | Liquids pass through the stomach too quickly to trigger fullness. Fruit requires chewing and takes longer to digest, allowing you to feel full. |
| ClifBar or PowerBar | ProtiDiet, Pure Protein, Atkins Advantage, or ZonePerfect protein bars | ClifBars and PowerBars (among other brands) contain mostly carbohydrate, which will drive up blood sugar and insulin, causing rebound hunger. They may be great for athletes who need quick sources of energy, but they're not great for overeaters. The other options are high in protein to slow digestion and induce fullness. |
| Most cold breakfast cereals (especially those with added sugar) | All-Bran, Bran Buds, Raisin Bran (⅓ cup) | High-fiber breakfast cereals digest more slowly, triggering a more lasting sense of fullness than lower-fiber cereals. |

# 5

# The Skinny Lunch Makeover

o you feel less hungry midmorning than you used to? Do you have more energy around noon than you used to? I bet you do. If you had tried to make over lunch before you made over breakfast, the change would be much harder. You'd be hungrier at lunch, so you'd have to use Navy Seal–like willpower to keep yourself away from sandwiches, wraps, and chips. Now, you're not as hungry and your cravings have probably subsided. You're ready.

## Why It Works

First, let's talk about the importance of lunch. Fewer of my patients skip lunch than breakfast, but some do. Usually these lunch skippers have one of two mind-sets. Some get really busy at work and forget to eat lunch, in which case they compensate in the late afternoon by raiding the vending machine. Others are members of the Meal Skippers Dieting Club. They firmly believe that skipping meals helps them consume fewer calories, even though this dieting method has failed—time and time again—to ever work.

Once again, when you skip lunch, you often end up gaining weight rather than losing it. Going more than five hours between meals causes hunger hormones to rise and fullness hormones to drop. When you eventually eat—after seven or eight hours of not eating—you overeat, consuming far more calories than you would had you simply sat down to two meals rather than one. This time span between meals also turns on a fat-storage switch. Your brain turns down metabolism, getting your muscles to conserve calories, and a higher percentage of the calories you consume at dinner go straight to your fat cells.

When fourteen young women taking part in a Netherlands study consumed three meals a day (breakfast, lunch, and dinner), their bodies burned more fat over twenty-four hours, compared to when they consumed just two daily meals. The women also reported feeling more satisfied, despite the fact that they consumed the same number of calories in both conditions.

## How to Do It

You'll start lunch with salad, then vegetables, and then lean protein. I can't quote you many studies to prove that eating foods in this order works. I can only tell you that I've been recommending that my patients eat this way since the mid-1990s, and they consistently report that it helps them stop eating before they've overeaten.

Here's how each of these courses affects your appetite.

**Salad:** Since the day that the salad was invented, foodies have argued whether it should be served first or last. Medical practitioners such as Hippocrates and Galen believed that "raw vegetables easily slipped through the system" and, as a result, were an ideal first course. Other Greeks and Romans believed that the vinegar used in salad dressing destroyed the taste of the wine, so salad should be served last. As it turns out, Hippocrates was right, but not for the right reasons. Salad is an ideal first course precisely because it does *not* slip through the system, as he believed. Salad takes up room in the stomach and intestines and slows digestion, filling you up on almost no calories. Consider how much of the following foods you can eat and for how few calories:

- 2 cups lettuce = 15 calories
- An entire bell pepper = 30 calories

- One large cucumber = 34 calories
- 1 cup mushrooms = 15 calories
- 1 cup broccoli = 30 calories

These vegetables are also heavy foods. We tend to think of heavy foods as cream based, but cream-based foods are actually light in weight. A cup of so-called heavy cream weighs down your stomach with 238 grams and sets you back 821 calories. That cucumber weighs down your stomach even more, with 280 grams, but for only 34 calories. Penn State's Dr. Barbara Rolls, the author of the popular book *Volumetrics,* has called this measurement "calorie density." She's shown that foods with a low calorie density (few calories per gram) are more filling, calorie for calorie, than high-calorie-density foods (many calories per gram).

Most vegetables are low in calorie density. Why are they so heavy? In a word, water. Ninety percent of that cucumber is water. This is true for nearly all vegetables, and, when water comes embedded inside food, it weighs it down and adds no calories.

This water weight dramatically reduces your appetite. In one of Dr. Rolls's studies, when forty-two women consumed salad as a first course, they ate 7 to 12 percent less pasta than when they had no salad. So if you consume the more filling foods first, you'll have less room for the less filling foods later, and they won't have as much of an adverse impact on your feelings of hunger and satiety.

All salads are not equally filling. To fill up on fewer calories, your salad

· · · · · · · · · · · · · · · · · · · · · · · · · · · · · · · · · · · · · · · · · · · · · ·

## The Skinny on . . . Why Vinegar Reduces Appetite

Not only does vinegar spoil the taste of wine, it also spoils your appetite. If you add vinegar to salad dressing, it will help slow digestion of everything else you eat. Arizona State University researchers determined that vinegar slowed the entrance of glucose into the bloodstream by 55 percent, especially when study participants consumed rapidly digested carbohydrate foods such as bagels. The more acetic acid in your vinegar, the more it slows the blood sugar response. Choose white, cider, or balsamic vinegar. Because they are made with vinegar, fermented and pickled products also slow digestion, which is why pickles can be great craving soothers.

must be nutrient dense but *not* calorie dense. Toppings such as croutons, cheese, fried tortilla strips, bacon, and creamy full-fat dressing drive up the calorie density of salad, and interestingly, this seems to induce hunger rather than fullness. When Rolls's study participants ate energy-dense salads with creamy dressings and lots of cheese, they ate between 8 and 17 percent *more* pasta (145 calories) than when they had no appetizer at all. Why? Because most of the calories in the salad were fattening; they triggered more hunger and didn't trigger enough fullness.

**Vegetables:** Like your salad, vegetables are low in calories, rich in nutrients, filled with water, and relatively heavy. They take a long time to eat, so they slow your eating pace. They contain fiber to slow digestion, and, with the exceptions of corn and potatoes (which are really starches), they are universally low on the glycemic load scale (see chapter 13 for the glycemic loads of many different foods).

**Skinny Solution:** I don't recommend you eat sandwiches on this plan, but I know how it goes. There will be times when a sandwich is either your only option or the only food you really want to eat. In that case, choose the highest-fiber whole-grain bread available and the smallest serving of bread. If you normally get a 12-inch sub, try a 6-inch one instead and have a salad first. Even better, have a sandwich with sliced bread instead of a hoagie roll, which cuts the starch even more. Try light bread, and, if possible, eat it open faced.

Like the salad, vegetables help fill you up on fewer calories. In a Penn State study of 71 women, participants who increased their consumption of vegetables as they cut fat reduced more daily calories, lost more weight, and reported less hunger than another group of women who only cut fat and did not try to increase their vegetable intake.

**Lean protein:** By the time you get to your lean protein, you will have already consumed at least 2 cups of food. Consider that your stomach is roughly the size of an eggplant and you can easily see how this eating approach improves your sense of fullness. Lean protein continues to fill you up because it requires lots of chewing, which slows your eating pace and provides more time for those fullness signals from your stomach and intestines to reach your brain. It's also, as I've mentioned, the most satisfying and appetite suppressing of all of the nutrients. Because you are choosing lean options, you can consume a hearty portion of protein, too. Remember that 5 ounces of skinless chicken breast has only 230 calories. The same amount of chicken fried—with all that fat and starchy breading—brings you to 370 calories, 50 percent more. More important, the fried breading contains the qualities of—you guessed it—fattening foods.

Try to eat lunch in the following order.

## Appetizer

Start with a salad made with *at least* 1 cup vegetables. You can consume as much salad as you want on this plan. It's an all-you-can-eat option, so don't skimp. Many of my patients have found that they feel most satisfied if this portion of the meal is at least 3 cups, and Penn State research shows that doubling the size of your premeal salad from 1½ cups salad to 3 cups salad helps you eat about 100 fewer calories during the rest of the meal. Make your salad with any combination of your favorite greens and/or vegetables.

Dress the salad with 1 to 2 teaspoons olive oil and all the vinegar you like, 1 to 2 tablespoons commercially prepared vinaigrette, or 2 tablespoons reduced-fat or light dressing. You can also choose from the homemade salad dressings described in chapter 12. Serve your salad on a plate instead of in a bowl. It looks like more food, so you'll feel more satisfied.

## Vegetable Side Dish

Eat your side dish before your main course, if possible. Consume at least 1 cup steamed vegetables, such as broccoli, cauliflower, zucchini, green beans, spinach, cabbage, Brussels sprouts, asparagus, tomatoes, eggplant,

. . . . . . . . . . . . . . . . . . . . . . . . . . . . . . . . . . . . . . . . .

**Skinny Solution:** If you feel ravenous at the start of lunch and, as a result, find yourself marching to the office cafeteria for some fatty comfort food rather than the skinny meal you packed in your bag, I have an easy solution: eat lunch earlier than usual. You're hungry because you are going too long between meals, especially if you eat breakfast very early in the morning. Having lunch at 11:30 or noon instead of 12:30 or 1:00 P.M. can make all the difference.

mushrooms, and carrots. Yes, I did include carrots on that list. Many years ago, some diets cautioned against eating carrots because of their carbohydrate content, particularly when cooked. But the carbohydrate in carrots dramatically affects blood sugar only if you eat a lot of carrots. For example, you'd have to eat ½ pound or 6 medium carrots to total 50 grams, the amount of carbohydrate needed to raise blood sugar significantly. That's a lot. Most people don't eat anywhere near that much, and when the blood sugar response of carrots is calculated based on a typical portion size, they fall to the low end on the glycemic load scale.

## Main Course

Finish lunch with at least 5 ounces lean protein. If you are a large man, you may need a larger portion of protein to feel satisfied. You can increase this portion up to 8 ounces if needed. You may use any main-course recipe in chapter 12 or these lean-protein options:

- Skinless chicken breast
- Skinless turkey breast
- Water-packed tuna
- Tuna or chicken salad, made with 1 tablespoon reduced-fat mayonnaise
- Any canned fish, shellfish, or sardines water-packed
- 2 soy or turkey burger patties without a roll

As you progress to Phase 2, you may add a high-fiber starch at the end of the meal. Eat the starch only if you are hungry, eat it only at the end of the meal, and hold it to one of the following portion sizes:

- 1 slice whole-grain bread (at least 3 grams of fiber per slice)
- 2 slices light whole-grain bread (at least 1.5 grams of fiber per slice)
- 1 slice rye or pumpernickel bread
- Half of a whole-wheat pita
- 1 mini whole-wheat pita
- 1 Thomas' Light Multi Grain English muffin (8 grams of fiber!)

If you don't have this question swimming around in your head this very minute, it will pop up eventually. You'll eventually wonder: do I have to eat lunch in this three-step order every single day? No, you don't.

You can certainly combine one or all of the steps by consuming a grilled chicken salad or a chicken-and-vegetable stir-fry. You can open a can of tuna, throw it on a bed of lettuce, and serve it with a side of baby carrots. Many of the main-course recipes in chapter 12 do just that, and you are free to use any of them as a lunch option.

## Fattening vs. Filling Foods

| Fattening Lunch Options | Filling Lunch Options | Why? |
|---|---|---|
| Huge salad loaded with croutons, cheese, and full-fat dressing | Huge salad loaded with chopped veggies and dressed with vinaigrette | High-calorie salad add-ons such as croutons and fatty dressings are easy to overeat. They also seem to trigger the desire to eat, so you consume more food at the next course. |
| 12-inch submarine sandwich with chips | 6-inch whole-grain submarine sandwich with double meat, extra lettuce and tomatoes, mustard and a little mayo, side salad, baby carrots | A 6-inch sub is just as filling as a 12-inch sub, but provides far fewer calories. The salad and baby carrots weigh down the stomach, inducing fullness for almost no calories. |
| Fast-food burger, fries, and soft drink | Side salad, grilled chicken cutlet or turkey burger patty, side of fruit | The quintessential fast-food meal will set you back more than 1,000 calories. It's loaded with trans fats, which tend to trigger hunger. They are also highly caloric, making them easy to overeat. The sugar in the soft drink travels through the stomach quickly, doing nothing to trigger fullness. The salad, chicken cutlet, and fruit, on the other hand, contain only about 400 calories, but they provide plenty of water, fiber, protein, and weight to turn off your appetite. You feel more satisfied even though you've consumed half as many calories. |

## Make It Happen

I can almost hear your thoughts: "I don't have time to chop veggies. I don't like veggies!" I'm with you. A cup of salad and a cup of side-dish vegetables is *a lot* of vegetables. Here are some easy ways to consume these vegetable servings without spending inordinate amounts of time standing in front of your chopping block:

- Purchase steam-in-a-bag vegetables, sold at most grocery stores. These are chopped and ready to eat. All you need to do is stick the bag in a microwave for a few minutes. Bring them with you to work. Some of my patients consume the entire bag, which often totals 2 to 3 cups vegetables. You'll find a list of recommended brands in chapter 13.
- Purchase any number of commercially prepared cut vegetables such as baby carrots, broccoli florets, and cauliflower florets. Bring them to work and eat them plain as a side dish or dip them in salsa, hummus, or one of the salad dressings in chapter 12.
- Stash cans of soup in your desk. Vegetable and bean soups count as one of your vegetable servings. When you are tired of eating lettuce, use a soup course as an appetizer. It's just as filling. Just make sure the soup does not contain rice, potatoes, or pasta.
- Get Chinese takeout. Order steamed vegetables with chicken or shrimp. Get a double portion and eat half for lunch one day, and the other half the next. Just make sure to get the sauce on the side and use as little of it as possible (no more than 2 tablespoons). Chinese sauces are usually loaded with both sugar and fat.
- Eat last night's leftovers. You haven't yet made over dinner, but once you do, you'll be consuming lots of salad and vegetable side dishes at that meal as well. Whenever you are making vegetables, double or triple the portion so you have leftovers to use in your lunch bag. Whenever you eat out, ask for a double or triple portion of vegetables. Box up the remainder and eat them for lunch the following day.
- Use bagged lettuce to make salads. It saves time. Keep the lettuce in its original bag until you need it. When unopened, the

bag has been puffed up with nitrogen to protect the leaves. Once you open it, close it with a clip. The bag is designed to let the optimal amount of oxygen in and out, to lengthen the freshness of the greens, allowing them to last longer before they wilt. Dress your salad just before eating, and not when you assemble it at home. The dressing makes greens soggy, causing them to wilt.

- Get supermarket takeout. Head to the grocery store during your lunch break. Assemble your salad at the salad bar. In the frozen-food aisle, grab a frozen entrée, choosing from recommended brands in chapter 13. Mix ½ cup canned (rinsed and drained) chickpeas, kidney beans, or lean lunch meat into your frozen dinner to make it more filling.

- To keep things interesting, expand your repertoire of salads and vegetable side dishes. Use the recipes in chapter 12 for inspiration.

## Eating-Out Advice

I'm so sick of hearing about diets that tell people they can't eat out. I want to ask the authors of these plans, "Do you live in the real world?" Go ahead and eat out or order in. Just use this advice:

**Ask a lot of questions.** Get nutrition information before you go. Some seemingly "good" options are really fattening. Consider the following:

- Chili's Chicken Caesar Salad has 1,010 calories and 76 grams of fat
- Ruby Tuesday's Bella Turkey Burger has 1,145 calories and 71 grams of fat
- On the Border's Blackened Chicken Fiesta Salad has 1,150 calories and 75 grams of fat
- Romano's Macaroni Grill Chicken Caesar Salad has 920 calories and 69 grams of fat

Those are not skinny options! Extra fat and/or sugar has been added to these dishes to put them over the top in terms of calories. When ordering a salad, pay careful attention to the add-ons. Croutons, bacon bits, bacon, cheese, raisins, nuts, and creamy full-fat dressings drive up the calorie content. Pick just one high-calorie topping for your salad. It's okay to splurge on nuts, a creamy dressing, cheese, or croutons, but only splurge once. Keep the rest of the salad lean. If you can't modify the salad when you order it, then modify it when it comes to the table. If there is a huge amount of cheese, take half of it off. The same goes for nuts, croutons, raisins, and other high-calorie add-ons.

Use these additional salad-ordering tips:

- Make sure the meat that comes with your salad is skinless, not breaded, and not fried.
- Bring your own dressing, ask for low-calorie dressing, or get the dressing on the side and use as little of it as possible.

**Always get sauce on the side.** Sauces add fat and sugar to your meal, increasing the caloric content but doing nothing to fill you up. If anything, they may prolong hunger. Consider the calories in the following sauces:

- 2 tablespoons aioli = 195 calories
- ¼ cup béarnaise = 220 calories
- 1 pat butter = 35 calories
- 2 tablespoons butter sauce = 205 calories
- 2 tablespoons hollandaise sauce = 185 calories
- 1 tablespoon pesto sauce = 155 calories
- ¾ cup Chinese brown sauce = 122 calories
- ¾ cup Chinese black bean sauce = 174 calories

I recommend the following eating-out options for lunch:

**Chinese:** (1) Hot and sour soup. (2) Steamed chicken, shrimp, or tofu with any of the following vegetables: steamed or lightly sautéed broccoli, snowpeas, spinach, eggplant, peppers, asparagus, mushrooms, water chestnuts, and ginger. Eat the vegetables first.

**Japanese:** (1) Seaweed salad or regular salad. (2) Edamame. (3) Sashimi, teriyaki chicken or fish, or broiled (yakimono) tuna or salmon.

**Mexican:** (1) Salad. (2) Chicken or shrimp fajitas without the tortilla. Eat the veggies first.

**Italian:** (1) Grilled vegetable antipasti or salad. (2) Steamed spinach (Florentine), broccoli rabe with garlic, roasted red peppers, or roasted eggplant. (3) Broiled fish or chicken piccata, marsala, marinara, arrabbiata, or cacciatore.

**Wendy's:** Grilled chicken Caesar salad, grilled chicken salad, mandarin chicken salad, taco salad, or side salad with small chili. Eliminate croutons, noodles, taco chips, or sour cream that may come with the salads.

**McDonald's:** Bacon ranch salad with grilled chicken, Caesar salad with grilled chicken, California Cobb salad with grilled chicken. Ask for Newman's Own low-fat balsamic vinaigrette or low-fat family recipe Italian dressing.

**Subway:** "Under 6 grams of fat" salads—ham, chicken, turkey breast, or veggie delite.

# 6

# The Skinny Snack Makeover

David seemed to be following the *Skinny* food plan without fail, but he still reported excessive hunger in the evening. He continually found himself overeating at dinner and beyond, and he didn't know why. When we went over his food records, I noticed he ate the same afternoon snack nearly every day. It was a candy bar.

When I asked him about it, he told me that the only available snacks at work came from a vending machine. "I know I should pack snacks and bring them with me, but I never get around to it," he admitted.

"I think the candy bar is what's making you so hungry at night," I said. "It's setting you back 300 calories, but it's 300 calories of sugar and fat that does nothing to fill you up. You might feel full temporarily after eating it, but the hunger soon returns."

"I don't have any other options," he said.

"Does that vending machine have bags of nuts?" I asked.

He thought for a moment. "Yes, I think it does."

"Have the nuts," I told him. The nuts contained roughly the same number of calories as the candy bar, but they were filling, whereas the candy bar was fattening. The nuts allowed him to eat less later on in the evening. This one simple switch got him past a weight-loss plateau.

## Why It Works

Midmorning and midafternoon snacks act as mini appetite suppressants. It takes your body three to five hours to process the food you eat, and, interestingly, it takes your body roughly the same amount of time to digest a huge meal as a small one. In some cases larger meals digest even more quickly than smaller ones, causing earlier and more intense spikes in hunger. As a result, most people feel more satisfied and less hungry when they eat one to two snacks and somewhat smaller meals than when they eat huge meals, but no snacks.

If you don't snack and go too long without eating, blood sugar drops too low. You feel tired. Sugar cravings increase, and your hunger levels go through the roof. You can't stop thinking about food, and the food you can't stop thinking about is usually fattening. It's loaded with starch, fat, sugar, or all three. Once you start eating these types of foods, you want to eat even more. You feel hungrier with each additional bite, and you keep eating and eating and eating. That's why it's important to snack *before* you feel hungry.

## Fattening Snacks vs. Filling Snacks

You may be scratching your head and thinking to yourself, "I thought snacking caused weight gain." You're right. It can, but only if you snack at the wrong times of day, and on the wrong types of foods.

What is the wrong time of day for a snack? In two words: after dinner. People who gain weight from snacking usually do so because they eat very little during the day, and then can't stop eating after dinner. They skip breakfast, eat a very small lunch, and forgo snacks during the afternoon. By the time they get home, they are ravenous and the snacking starts. They nibble as they prepare dinner. They eat as they set the table. They eat as they are walking food dishes to the table. They eat first and second helpings. Then they nibble off the plates as they clear the table and clean the kitchen. They snack all night long, and they consume far more calories after dinner than most people consume in three square meals.

This is not the type of snacking I recommend. Rather, I want you to snack *before* you feel hungry. Have an optional snack midmorning, if you need one. Everyone should consider a midafternoon snack.

Now, let's talk about the right and wrong types of snacks. Fattening snacks, unfortunately, are what most people tend to snack on. They are candy bars, snack chips, cookies, soft drinks, and the assortment of sweet and salty foods you find in air-puffed bags in the middle aisle of the grocery store.

These high-sugar, high-starch, high-fat snacks start a vicious cycle in which hunger creates more hunger, and a little snacking turns into a lot of snacking. Have you ever felt hungry, jittery, or sleepy within a few hours of snacking? It's because you ate a hunger-promoting snack. Once you start, you're hungry again, and you are craving sweets, so you reach for another snack.

Fattening snacks also tend to house addictive flavors or textures. Sweet and salty flavors tend to make

you want to eat more, and most processed snack chips, cookies, and cakes contain both flavors. So does the texture combination of sugar with fat. That's why you can't stop at a reasonable portion. You may tell yourself that you're going to have just three chips or just one cookie, but it rarely works out that way. What about those portion-controlled 100-calorie snack packs that you see increasingly at the grocery store? Most of these snacks are fattening, too. Yes, they contain only 100 calories, but they also make you hungrier, making you want to reach for another snack or overeat at dinner.

So what's the point of snacking? Unlike fattening snacks, filling snacks help you eat less at subsequent meals. They contain fiber, protein, or both. These nutrients slow digestion and stabilize blood sugar, among other things.

To understand the difference between filling and fattening snacks, consider a study done in Australia. Researchers there fed twenty-three women a high-protein/high-fiber snack bar or a similar bar that was high in fat and refined (quickly digesting) carbohydrate (similar in composition to your everyday bag of potato chips). A few hours later, the researchers placed the women in the equivalent of a dieter's worst nightmare. They offered them an all-you-can-eat buffet. What do you think happened? The women who'd snacked on the high-protein/high-fiber bars had more self-control than the ones who had the high-fat, high-carbohydrate bars, and, as a result, they consumed 5 percent less from the buffet, a savings of 70 calories. Their blood sugar and insulin levels were also lower during the nine hours after the snack, keeping their energy levels steady.

## How to Do It

On this plan, you'll consume filling snacks. Rich in protein and/or fiber, they provide true staying power.

You may consume up to two snacks a day.

**Midmorning snack:** This snack is optional. Not everyone needs it. If you eat breakfast at 8 and lunch at noon, you may not feel hungry midmorning because you're going only four hours between those meals. If you are an early breakfast eater—you eat around 6 A.M.—you'll probably find that you are hungry again around 10. If so, have a midmorning snack.

**Midafternoon snack:** This snack is mandatory. For most people, the span between lunch and dinner is at least seven hours. That's too long, given that the body clears your lunch in three to five hours. Without a midafternoon snack, most people are too hungry at dinner and tend to lose control.

Consume your snack before you feel ravenously hungry. If you normally feel hungry at 4:30 P.M., for example, consume your afternoon snack at 4. This provides you with more self-control.

Choose snacks that are high in protein and/or fiber and that are no more than 100 calories. Great options include the following:

**Fruit:** Fruit is high in fiber, water, and weight and low in calories and sugar. One cup of blueberries, for example, contains only 83 calories, but it fills you up with 3.5 grams of fiber and 122 grams of water. Fruit is also packed with wholesome nutrition. The antioxidants in berries, for example, help prevent cancer and stroke, and they keep the memory sharp.

It's important to eat whole fruit—complete with the skin and seeds— and not fruit products such as applesauce, fruit juice, or canned fruit. Most of the fiber in fruit lies in the skin. Once you remove the skin, fruit becomes much less filling. Mashing up the fruit into a sauce makes it less filling still, because the GI tract does not have to work as hard to digest sauce as it does to digest whole fruit.

Once again, work by Penn State researcher Dr. Barbara Rolls bears this out. She and her colleagues fed volunteers one of three snacks, all of which contained the same number of calories: an apple, applesauce, and apple juice. When study volunteers ate the apple fifteen minutes before lunch, they consumed an average of 187 fewer calories during lunch than when they consumed applesauce, drank apple juice, or ate nothing at all just before this meal. All the snacks were made out of apples, but the solid fibrous one cut food intake; the other forms of the apple did not.

**Nuts:** Although they have been blamed for leading to weight gain, nuts, when consumed in reasonable portions, can actually help control weight. One ounce of almonds, for instance, provides 5 grams of appetite-suppressing protein and 4 grams of appetite-suppressing fiber. People who munched on 500 calories' worth of cocktail nuts daily for an eight-week-long Purdue University study didn't gain any weight. Researchers suspect that the nuts were so filling that participants ate less throughout the rest of the day without even realizing it.

The type of fat in nuts may also be good for your overall health. In the ongoing Nurses' Health Study of 86,000 women done at Brigham and Women's Hospital in Boston and at the Harvard School of Public Health, women who ate more than 5 ounces of nuts per week had one-third as many heart attacks as women who never or rarely ate nuts. Choose only raw or dry-roasted nuts. Oil-roasted nuts are fried in oil, which adds about 10 percent more fat, often fat that is saturated or hydrogenated.

**Soup:** It's not something you typically think of as a snack food, but it's a powerful appetite suppressant. When twenty-four women taking part in a Penn State study ate three different snacks containing the same ingredients—a chicken rice casserole, chicken rice casserole with a glass of water, or chicken rice soup—they reported less hunger and ate 80 fewer calories at a subsequent meal when they ate the soup versus when they ate the other two snacks.

**Vegetables:** I'm sure that I'm starting to sound like a broken record. Vegetables are unlimited on this plan, so if you are a big snacker who needs to work on portion control, vegetables are a great option because you can snack on them all afternoon long.

**Cheese and yogurt:** Cheese sticks and small yogurt and cottage cheese containers come in convenient individual portions for snacking. Cheese is low in carbohydrate and rich in appetite-suppressing protein. One cup of cottage cheese, for example, offers 14 grams of protein.

**Edamame:** Nearly 40 percent of the calories in edamame comes from protein (11 grams per ½ cup), making soybeans higher in protein than other beans and even some animal products. They are also rich in fiber, with 5 grams per ½ cup.

Use the following snack choices. Choose one or two a day:

1 cup fresh berries or melon cubes
½ grapefruit
1 whole apple, nectarine, or plum
6 to 12 almonds or cashews, 10 to 20 small peanuts, or 4 to 8 walnut halves
4 ounces 1% cottage cheese
8 ounces low-fat artificially sweetened yogurt (90 to 120 calories per container)
½ cup fat-free, sugar-free pudding (made from the mix, not the premade snack cup)
⅔ cup edamame
Unlimited amount of raw vegetables
2 wedges Laughing Cow Light Cheese on 2 celery sticks
1 cup carrot or celery sticks with 2 tablespoons hummus
1 sliced apple with 2 teaspoons peanut butter
1 pear and 5 whole cashews
1 ounce part-skim mozzarella cheese and 4 Triscuits
½ cup 1% cottage cheese with cinnamon and 4 walnut halves
1 ounce reduced-fat cheddar cheese with 1 cup fresh berries

½ cup 1% cottage cheese topped with 1 sliced kiwi and cinnamon

8 ounces artificially sweetened yogurt and 1½ tablespoons trail mix

12 ounces nonfat café latte sprinkled with cinnamon and 6 almonds on the side

1 Ryvita or Wasa cracker with 1 cup canned ready-to-serve bean soup, Lentil Soup (page 184), Easiest Vegetable Soup (page 183), Gazpacho (page 184), or Tuscan White Bean Soup (page 188)

1 cup salad greens with ¼ cup each chickpeas and kidney beans, with 1 tablespoon vinaigrette

## Make It Happen

Skinny snacking requires planning and preparation. If you're like David and have access to a vending machine that supplies nuts or some other skinny snack, great. Most people don't, however. The best way to make sure you eat at least every three to five hours is to have plenty of healthful foods for meals and snacks available to you at all times, including nuts, fruits, vegetables, whole grains, and low-fat dairy products.

Use these pointers:

**Portion your snacks carefully.** Portion your snacks into small zip-top bags that you can stash in your cabinet or in your desk at work. *Don't* reach your hand into a large container of nuts and assume that you'll stop eating automatically. Your brain isn't that good at measuring portion sizes when it sees a big portion of snack food. My colleague at Cornell University Dr. Brian Wansink demonstrated that most people will overeat large snack portions even when the snack doesn't taste good. In a study of 158 moviegoers, participants consumed 33 percent more popcorn from a large container than from a medium container, even though the popcorn was fourteen days old and incredibly stale.

**Plan your snacks.** Most people make unhealthy snack choices in the moment, when they are hungry. If you have a healthy snack with you, you'll more likely eat a filling snack when you need it. Stock your fridge—at home and/or at work—with fresh fruits and vegetables, low-fat dairy foods such as cottage cheese and yogurt, and raw nuts, so you can easily grab something when it's time for you to eat. Stash some quick and tasty snacks in your desk drawer, too.

## Fattening vs. Filling Foods

| Fattening Snack Options | Filling Snack Options | Why? |
|---|---|---|
| Planters Tubes | Planters Single-Serve bags | Planters Tubes are deceptive. They look like a small serving of nuts, but they actually provide two servings, totaling about 250 calories. Research shows that most people can't eat half a container and stop. The single-serving bags, on the other hand, contain a more ideal serving, so you eat less automatically. |
| Apple juice | Apple | A whole apple takes a long time to eat, contains fiber, and takes a long time to digest. You can drink apple juice much more quickly. It's not as heavy as an apple and it contains no fiber, so it does not flip your fullness switch. |
| 100-calorie snack pack, any variety | Small individual container of 2% cottage cheese | The cottage cheese and the 100-calorie snacks contain roughly the same number of calories, and they are both portioned for you. But the cottage cheese contains protein to fill you up. The snack packs offer no nutritional value, and most contain sugar, starch, and fat that triggers rebound hunger. |

# 7

# The Skinny Dinner Makeover

Dinner and the hours afterward usually mark the time of day that most people lose control, especially when they follow typical calorie-controlled diets. A USDA survey found, for example, that most people consume about 42 percent of their total day's calories at dinner and beyond, with overweight adults consuming significantly more calories at dinner than slimmer adults.

Eating huge portions at dinner sets you up for weight gain for a number of reasons. First, you feel less satisfied when you consume large amounts of food at night than you do when you consume them earlier in the day. In a study of more than 800 men and women done at Sam Houston University in Huntsville, Texas, study participants who fueled up with a large breakfast of any type—high in protein, high in fat, or high in carbohydrate—tended to eat fewer overall calories during a typical day than people who ate a small breakfast but a large dinner. Other research from the same institution shows that postmeal fullness and satisfaction tends to decrease later in the day compared to earlier. A big breakfast controls appetite long term. A big dinner? Not so much, and it may even cause you to feel hungrier the next day.

Research also shows that your body more effectively burns off calories consumed earlier in the day than later in the day. When USDA researchers put ten women on two diets, one with 70 percent of calories consumed at breakfast and another with 70 percent of calories consumed at dinner, the large-breakfast eaters lost more weight than the large-dinner eaters, even though they consumed the same number of daily calories.

So it makes sense to fill up with a large breakfast and end the day with a more moderate dinner. Here's the challenge: getting yourself to actually do it. I'm sure you've already tried to put an end to overeating at dinner and afterward many times. My patients have told me stories of the promises they'd made to themselves before switching over to the *Skinny* lifestyle. They'd promised, "No more late-night snacks. The kitchen is closed at seven P.M." Then, after work, they'd find themselves in the car, on their way home, their resolve already faltering. They'd pull into the driveway, and their resolve would crumble even more. Then they'd walk into the kitchen and the eating would start. After dinner, the true cravings hit and they found themselves hitting the chips, ice cream, and cookies. Whatever calorie control they'd managed to impose during the day had been undone by the end of the evening.

This plan is not about willpower. It's about using the latest science to allow your body to sense how many extra calories you have stored and to utilize those, rather than order out for more. That's the power of this plan. Now that you've switched about 70 percent of your eating over to *Skinny* meals, I'm guessing that you are noticing some differences at the dinner table. Perhaps you're not quite as ravenous when you sit down at the table. Perhaps you no longer reach for seconds or no longer snack as much after the meal's end. That's *The Skinny* at work. Making over breakfast enabled you to make over lunch, which enabled you to make over your snacks, which now enables you to make over dinner.

To feel satisfied on fewer calories at dinner and beyond, you need follow only two rules:

**Serve yourself huge portions of filling foods and much smaller portions of fattening foods.** If you put 2 cups of mashed potatoes on your plate—even though you plan to eat only a few spoonfuls—you'll probably end up eating 2 cups of mashed potatoes. Dr. Rolls's studies show that the mere sight of large portions increases eating by nearly 40 percent, or about 273 calories per meal.

Go ahead and dish yourself huge portions of filling foods such as salad and vegetables. The more of these foods you see and eat, the better. Keep a huge bowl of salad on the table, in plain sight. Keep a huge bowl of steamed vegetables there, too. Have as many seconds of either as you want.

On the other hand, do control the amount of starchy, sugary, and other fattening foods you put on the table. Plate these foods in the kitchen, keeping their serving bowls out of sight. If you feel especially tempted to go back to the kitchen for sec-

onds, ask everyone in your family to dish up their starch servings, and then store the remainder in the refrigerator before you sit down to eat. You'll be much less tempted to break into a covered container of cold pasta than you would a hot bowl sitting on the countertop.

**Eat filling foods first.** When Dr. Rolls fed twenty-three university students filling foods such as salad, soup, and vegetables first, they ate less of subsequent courses, no matter how large the portions of the fattening foods sitting in front of them. Consuming filling foods first, she and her research team found, can shrink appetite by 24 percent, enough to cause you to eat about 575 fewer daily calories. Eat fattening foods only if you still feel hungry after eating filling foods. By consuming huge portions of low-calorie, filling foods such as salad and vegetables first, you'll be less likely to want to eat hunger-promoting foods such as starch and dessert. In this way, you'll feel more satisfied and consume fewer overall calories, without willing yourself to eat less.

Here's how each course helps fill you up on fewer calories.

**Appetizer:** You'll fill up on foods that are low in calories but heavy in weight, high in volume, and/or rich in appetite-suppressing protein. You can choose up to three appetizers. They include the following:

- *Salad.* As you learned when you made over lunch, salad is packed with low-calorie, slow foods that are rich in appetite-suppressing fiber, water, and weight. Salads take a long time to eat and require a lot of chewing, which helps instill a sense of satisfaction. Eating a salad before dinner can help reduce your total food intake by 12 percent.

- *Soup.* Most vegetable- or bean-based soups are low in calories and high in satisfaction. A cup of vegetable soup, for example, sets you back only 81 calories, lentil soup just 120 calories, and gazpacho about 70. In Rolls's study of 60 men and women, study participants who consumed soup ate 20 percent less.
- *Shrimp or seafood cocktail.* Both are relatively high in appetite-suppressing protein, heavy with water, and low in calories. For example, 3 ounces of peeled cooked shrimp delivers 22 grams of protein, 56 grams of water, and just 116 calories. The same amount of lump crabmeat offers 17 grams of protein, 64 grams of water, and just 84 calories.

**Side dish:** Your vegetable side dish at dinner suppresses appetite for the same reason it does at lunch. The vegetables are low in calories, rich in nutrients, filled with water, and relatively heavy. They take a long time to eat, so they slow your eating pace. They contain fiber to slow digestion, and, with the exceptions of corn and potatoes, they are universally low on the glycemic load scale.

**Main course:** Lean protein helps at dinner for the same reason it does so at lunch. First, it takes some chewing, so it slows your eating pace, providing more time for those fullness signals from your stomach and intestines to reach your brain. It's also the most satisfying and appetite suppressing of all of the nutrients.

**High-fiber whole grain:** The fiber in whole grains slows the absorption of sugar into the bloodstream, inducing a long-lasting sense of fullness.

Most people eat dinner in the opposite order. They start with an alcoholic drink and starch, usually bread. When consumed before a meal on an empty stomach, alcohol is a true aperitif—it stimulates appetite. Your body metabolizes it first, before everything else you eat. The alcohol consumes blood sugar as it's metabolized, and a small drop in blood sugar signals your brain that it's time to eat, making you hungrier. One study found that an alcoholic drink before dinner increased eating by 15 percent.

Bread is just as problematic. The refined starch stimulates appetite, making you hungrier. Why do you think a restaurant, a business that makes money off selling food, gives you a free basket of bread when you arrive? It's not because they hope it will fill you up so you order less. They do it because bread makes you hungrier and reduces your sense of fullness or satiety, so you'll order and eat more. So a drink followed by a roll first stimulates your appetite and then breaks down your sense of fullness so you can eat more. It makes sense if you run a restaurant, but not if you're trying to lose weight.

## How to Do It

Dinner works the same way as lunch. You'll start with an appetizer, move on to a vegetable side dish, and finish with lean protein. Here are some specifics.

1. Start your meal with a salad (unlimited vegetables dressed with 1 to 2 teaspoons olive oil and vinegar, 1 to 2 tablespoons vinaigrette or reduced-fat dressing, or 1 serving of a dressing recipe in chapter 12), soup (clear broth, lentil, gazpacho, or vegetable without noodles or rice), and/or shrimp or seafood cocktail. You may have one, two, or all three of these options, depending on your appetite. Your salad should contain at least 1 cup vegetables and greens, and ideally 2 or 3 cups. You'll find numerous recipes for soup and salad first courses in chapter 12.
2. Have at least 1 cup nonstarchy vegetables. Choose from the list of recommended vegetables in chapter 13 and use the vegetable side-dish recipes in chapter 12 for inspiration.
3. Choose any of the main-course recipes in chapter 12 or have 5 to 8 ounces skinless chicken breast, fish, turkey breast, a soy or turkey burger, lean beef (London broil, filet mignon, flank steak), veal, pork tenderloin, or fresh baked ham. I recommend you consume red meat no more than twice a week. Although many types of red meat are just as lean as poultry or fish, most people tend to either supersize red meat portions, consuming more than this plan recommends, or choose fattier cuts than recommended.
4. At the end of the meal—after you've consumed everything else—you may have a ½-cup serving of a high-fiber grain or beans such as brown rice, wild rice, pasta, sweet potato, barley,

**Skinny Solution:** If you choose to have an alcoholic drink, have it with the main course, when it is least likely to affect your appetite. When you have alcohol with food, its appetite-stimulating effect is blunted. Please note that some people have a difficult time losing weight if they drink. If you make all of the changes that this program suggests and you have not reached your goal weight, *then* it's time to think about cutting back further with alcohol. Consume alcohol just once or twice a week or less often rather than every day.

. . . . . . . . . . . . . . . . . . . . . . . . . . . . . . . . . . . . . . . . . .

or whole-wheat pasta. Measure this course carefully. Consume no more than ½ cup. On a typical 12-inch dinner plate, that's about one eighth of the plate. Fill half of your plate with veggies, ⅜ (roughly ¾ of the other half) with protein, and the small space that is left with starch.

5. (Optional) You may have the following foods for dessert: ½ cup fat-free, sugar-free pudding or gelatin (such as Hunt's premade or Jell-O brand) topped with 1 to 2 tablespoons Cool Whip for dessert. Count this as one of your snacks.

Ideally, eat your vegetables before you have your protein, but you can certainly create one-dish meals such as chicken-and-vegetable stir-fry, roasted chicken with vegetables, or even a chicken-and-vegetable soup.

## Make It Happen

We all have those days when we're running from one task to another, come home exhausted at 7 or 8 P.M., and have just one thought: "I don't feel like cooking." These are usually the days that unravel the best of intentions, causing you to order a pizza and eat half of it. To increase your resolve on the busiest and most stressful of days, I recommend you keep a few no-cook, filling staples on hand at all times:

- Bagged salad mix
- Steam-in-a-bag vegetables

- One or more *Skinny*-recommended frozen dinners (page 201 in chapter 13)

Most frozen dinners contain just 200 calories, and most people need at least 400 to feel satisfied. Have the dinner with at least 1 cup of fresh, steamed, or frozen vegetables to increase feelings of fullness, even if veggies are included in the dinner. You can mix beans or cooked chicken or another meat into the dinner for extra protein.

You also can and should get used to eating out. I live in New York City and I counsel many New Yorkers who eat one or two (or more!) meals per day in restaurants. If I told them they had to cook every meal at home and never eat out, I'd go out of business because I'd have so few patients. Because I counsel so many New Yorkers who eat out so often, I know that you can indeed eat out and still lose weight, as long as you consistently choose the following *Skinny* options.

**Skinny Mini:** Women in a University of Illinois study who ate two packaged dinners a day dropped 5 more pounds in eight weeks compared to women who tried to consume the same amount of calories but made their own meals.

## Skinny Restaurant Options

### Chinese
Hot and sour soup or chicken broth
Steamed chicken or shrimp vegetable and noodle soup (ask to leave out the noodles)
Steamed dumplings (limit to three)
Moo goo gai pan (chicken with sautéed vegetables)
Moo shu beef or chicken (no crêpes)
Steamed salmon or bass with ginger and scallions
Steamed chicken, shrimp, or bean curd (tofu) with any of these vegetables: steamed broccoli, snow peas, spinach, eggplant, peppers, asparagus, mushrooms, water chestnuts, and ginger
To decrease calories, limit sauce to 2 to 3 tablespoons.

## Indian

Look for entrées cooked with tomatoes, onions, peppers, beans, lentils, spinach, and assorted spices or marinated in yogurt. Do not order vindaloo, korma, or biryani dishes, as they are high-fat selections!

Chicken or lentil soup
Vegetable, shrimp, or chicken kebabs
Tandoori chicken
Chana masala (chickpeas in tomato sauce)
To decrease calories, limit sauce to 2 to 3 tablespoons.

## Thai

Tom yum goong—hot and sour lemongrass broth with shrimp, bell peppers, and mushrooms
Vegetable soup
Thai salad (dressing on the side)
Cucumber salad (limit ground peanuts)
Shrimp or squid salad
Yum nua—grilled sliced beef, onions, tomatoes, lettuce, and Thai herbs
Lemongrass pork chop—grilled pork chop marinated with lemongrass, garlic, and lime juice
Gai ta krai—chicken marinated with lemongrass and served over a bed of onions, mushrooms, sweet basil, and black bean sauce
Grilled seared salmon—salmon spiced with soybean, garlic, ginger sauce, and chili on a platter
Garlic shrimp—sautéed grilled shrimp with garlic, peppers, onions, and tomato shoots
Thai fish stew
Broccoli with Thai basil—broccoli sautéed with baby corn, Thai basil, and chili paste
Bean curd sheets—shiitake mushrooms, bamboo shoots, and bean curd wrapped with bean curd skin, seared and served on a bed of spinach topped with basil black bean sauce

## Italian

Mixed salad
Mozzarella and tomato salad

Grilled vegetable antipasti
Sautéed spinach or broccoli rabe with garlic
Broiled fish or chicken
Broiled (not fried) chicken cutlet parmigiana
Grilled shrimp or scallops oreganato (other sauces)

## Japanese
Miso soup
Seaweed salad or salad with ginger dressing
Seared tuna or salmon
Edamame
Sashimi
Teriyaki chicken, fish, or beef
Negimaki
Chirashi

## Mexican
Black bean soup
Vegetarian or chicken chili
Salad with lettuce, pinto beans, black beans, salsa, and chicken or
    tuna with guacamole on the side (limit to 2 to 3 tablespoons)
Ceviche (fish marinated in lime juice and mixed with spices)
Chicken or shrimp fajitas with or without a soft whole-wheat
    tortilla
At Chipotle, order the Burrito Bowl with carnitas or chicken. Ask
    for light guacamole and cheese. Salsa is unlimited.

## Spanish
Chicken soup with chicken, carrots, onions, and lentils without
    rice, potatoes, and noodles
Grilled chicken with steamed beets, string beans, and carrots
Chicken, beef, or shrimp grilled or as kebabs
Boiled cassava with sautéed onions

## Steakhouse
House salad without croutons, with vinaigrette on the side
Lean cuts—London broil, filet mignon, round and flank steaks.
    Order petite cuts. Hold the butter.
Steamed vegetables without butter

Broiled chicken in white wine sauce
Broiled, grilled, charbroiled fish
Surf and turf without butter

## Subway

"Under 6 grams of fat" salads—ham, chicken, turkey breast, or
veggie delite

Any "under 6 grams of fat" sub on a 6-inch whole-wheat roll
with the bread scooped out. If you're hungry, have double meat
with extra lettuce and tomato on the 6-inch roll.

## Wendy's

Caesar salad with grilled chicken fillet, without croutons
Mandarin salad with grilled chicken fillet, without crispy noodles
Southwest taco salad without taco chips or sour cream
Side salad with chili
Dressings: reduced-fat creamy ranch, low-fat honey mustard,
Italian vinaigrette, ancho chipotle ranch dressing, or Caesar
dressing

## McDonald's

Choose any of the following salads without croutons and noodles.
You can also have any of the premium salads without chicken
and instead add 5 ounces of tofu, canned tuna or salmon, or
hard-boiled egg whites. Dress the salad with Newman's Own
low-fat dressing.

Premium southwest salad with grilled chicken
Premium Asian salad with grilled chicken
Premium bacon ranch salad with grilled chicken
Premium Caesar salad with grilled chicken

## Miscellaneous

Salad and soup combo
Greek salad
Fresh greens with salmon or tuna without mayonnaise
Grilled vegetable salad
Egg-white omelet with vegetables
Grilled or broiled chicken or fish with steamed vegetables

# Easy Time-Savers

Part of getting in the habit of consuming filling foods lies in learning how to cook them. Lean on the recipes in chapter 12 for help, along with the following advice.

**Make lots of chicken or turkey at once.** You can purchase cooked skinless chicken, or you can make your own once or twice a week. Purchase boneless, skinless chicken breasts in quantity and store them in the freezer in individual zip-top bags, so you can thaw one portion at a time. This way you'll always have chicken on hand for dinner. This is vitally important during those busy weeks when you don't have time to plan ahead. Once or twice a week, thaw a few breasts. Rinse them under cold water and pat them dry before cooking. Use one of the following cooking methods:

- Bake at 425°F for 10 to 15 minutes, or until the internal temperature of the chicken reaches 160°F.
- Poach in a deep skillet with 1 to 2 cups chicken broth. Bring the broth to a boil, reduce the heat, add the chicken, cover, and cook for 9 to 14 minutes, or until the internal temperature reaches 160°F.
- Grill over high heat for 8 to 10 minutes.

Refrigerate cooked chicken for three to four days.

If you're on a budget and can't afford to buy cooked chicken strips for salads, consider either buying an entire roasted chicken or roasting one once or twice a week. Cook at 400°F, breast side up, for 20 minutes, breast side down for another 20 minutes, and then breast side up for the final 20 minutes. Flipping the bird in this way will ensure that the chicken cooks evenly, resulting in more tender meat. Once you roast the bird, remove the skin and pull the meat off the bone (this is easier if the chicken is still warm). Store in a storage bag in the refrigerator for three to four days, using it on salads and other dishes.

**Always make more vegetables than you need.** Eat the leftovers for lunch the following day.

**Rely on convenience items.** Fresh and frozen vegetables are available in bags that you can stick directly in your microwave to steam. Consult the list of recommended brands on page 203 in chapter 13.

# How to Keep It Interesting

You'll be eating the same repertoire of foods when you start this plan. If you get sick of eating salad or chicken, use this advice.

**Skinny Mini:** Capsaicin, the active ingredient in cayenne and other hot peppers, may help you eat less by affecting levels of appetite-suppressing brain chemicals. Study participants who drank tomato juice spiked with red pepper consumed up to 16 percent fewer calories over two days than participants who had regular tomato juice.

**Try new foods.** Even if you don't think you like a particular vegetable, make it a few times anyway. Your taste buds change over time. Something you didn't like as a child may taste good when you're an adult.

**Try new recipes and cooking methods.** Try adding a new sauce, spice rub, marinade, or dressing. See chapter 12 for recipe ideas.

**Get creative with veggies.** Dice them up or purée them and add them to a sauce that you serve over your protein. Have them as part of a stir-fry. Try different cooking methods. Roast or grill them instead of steaming. Try cooking them in low-sodium chicken broth for extra flavor. Sprinkle your favorite spices over them, even if it's as simple as Mrs. Dash or another spice blend. Try sprinkling a little Parmesan cheese on top.

**Get creative with salads.** Many of our patients eventually tire of eating one to two salads a day. That's understandable. When you get bored with salad, try these ideas:

- Add more texture to your salads—for instance, by topping them with beans or avocado, or by using a different dressing.
- Have a leafless salad. Consult the salad recipes in chapter 12 for inspiration.

# How to Stay in Control

If, after switching to *Skinny* eating, you still find you are overeating at dinner and beyond, try this advice.

**Do something after dinner.** Get involved in something else to take the focus off food and eating. Sip a cup of hot tea, go for a walk, call a friend, play a board game with your family, or fire up the Wii Fit. Even brushing your teeth can serve as a nice finishing touch, and if you really want to keep yourself out of the kitchen, put whitening strips on your teeth.

**Snack on vegetables.** If you are chewing on baby carrots, you'll be less likely to sample higher-calorie fare instead.

**Ask someone else to clear the table.** Many of my patients tell me that cleanup is the toughest time because they continually find themselves sneaking bites of leftovers. Ask a family member to help clear the table, especially to scrape the plates and wrap up leftovers. You also may find it helpful to chew gum or nibble on raw vegetables as you clear the table.

**Make your own frozen dinners.** Many of my patients like to cook up a lot of food on the weekends, separate it into individual portions, and store those portions in the refrigerator or freezer. This way their dinner is already ready for them when they arrive home from work, and, thanks to the individual portion, there are no seconds to reach for.

**Eat in the dining room.** When study participants ate pizza just thirty minutes after a meal, they consumed 228 more calories from the pizza when they ate it in front of a TV instead of at a table with no distractions. Another U.K. study found that women who ate in front of the TV wanted to consume more food than women who ate in silence.

**Shift dinner time earlier.** Research shows that the longer the time gap between dinner and the previous meal, the more people tend to eat at dinner.

**Do all of the other meals right.** Usually when people have trouble at dinner, they still haven't completely made over the other meals. They may be eating too little for breakfast or skipping their afternoon snack. The most important way to eat less at night is to eat more earlier in the day.

**Think about why you are eating.** Are you eating out of hunger or for an emotional reason? This is where your food diary can really help. Whenever you find yourself reaching for seconds or snacking after dinner, write down what you ate, how you felt, and why you ate it. This can help you see if you are eating to relax, to celebrate, to socialize, or to distract yourself. In addition to hunger, you can also keep tabs on how your food tastes. The flavor of your food will diminish with each bite.

Try to stop eating when the flavor is at a 4 or 5, rather than waiting until it's at 0.

## What If You Slip Up?

Get right back on track. Few if any of my patients can claim that they've never cheated on a diet, and occasionally some really went off course, usually at night. It usually started with a dessert and went downhill from there. No matter how much of the wrong types of foods you consume at night, always get back on the plan in the morning. Think of breakfast not only as a way to break the fast, but also a way to break out of backsliding. Overeating at dinner is not the end of the world. Just get up and have protein for breakfast.

You will be hungrier the day after a splurge, and you'll have more cravings, too. But if you go ahead and eat starches and sweets for breakfast, you'll be hungrier later in the day. And if you eat badly then, you'll be hungrier for dinner. And the next morning, and so on. That's the cause of yo-yo dieting.

Break the cycle by getting up the morning after overindulging and getting right back on track by eating more protein than usual. You may feel hungrier than usual for one to three days, but the hunger will eventually subside and you'll be back on track.

# 8

# The Skinny Beverage Makeover

Kate's cardiologist referred her to my office. She weighed 190 pounds and was still gaining despite efforts to lose. The excess weight was nudging her blood sugar higher. If she didn't turn things around soon, she would develop diabetes.

"I don't understand," she said. "I don't eat anything. How can I keep gaining weight if I'm not eating anything?"

We looked over a food record that I asked Kate to keep for a week before the appointment. She was telling the truth. She was hardly eating anything. Based on the amount of food she consumed each day, she should have been losing, not gaining.

"What are you drinking?" I asked.

"Iced tea," she replied.

"How much?" I asked.

"I drink sixty-four ounces during a typical day. My mouth always feels dry, so I walk around with a glass and take sips whenever it feels dry." I knew her mouth probably felt dry because of her rising blood sugar levels coupled with some of the medications she was taking, but

I also suspected that the iced tea might be causing her weight to rise in the first place, contributing to the dryness.

"How many calories are in the tea?" I asked.

"What do you mean?" she said.

"The tea is probably sweetened with sugar," I explained. "It's adding unnecessary calories to your diet. It also might be making you hungrier."

"It's sugar free," she said.

"Are you certain?"

"Well, someone buys it for me, but I told them to get sugar free."

"Do me a favor and check."

After that appointment Kate checked the nutrition label on the bottle of tea that she usually drank. As it turned out, it was not sugar free. She did the math. Kate was consuming 640 calories of iced tea a day! She was shocked. No wonder she was gaining. When she switched from tea to water and began taking metformin to control her blood sugar, she lost 50 pounds.

## Why It Works

Carbonated soft drinks, fruit juice, coffee drinks, and alcohol account for 10 percent of calories in the American diet, and numerous studies have linked liquid calorie consumption with weight gain.

Consider the following:

- One study of 548 Massachusetts schoolchildren linked each additional daily soft drink with a 60 percent increased risk of obesity.
- The Harvard Nurses' Health Study determined that women who increased their consumption of sugar-sweetened beverages, such as sodas or fruit punch, from one per week to one or more per day consumed an average of 358 extra calories per day and gained a significant amount of weight over eight years. The women who reduced their intake of these beverages cut their daily calories by an average of 319 and gained less weight.
- A recent review of available studies conducted by researchers at Harvard determined that drinking one soft drink a day resulted in a 15-pound weight gain in a year.

Many people, like Kate, forget that calories from beverages count just as much as they do from food. They sip on beverages throughout the day, somewhat mindlessly, and at the end of the day they can't accurately recall how many of these beverages they've consumed.

Other people assume that some of these drinks are much less caloric than reality. For example, some people think sports drinks are low in calories. Well, they are lower in calories than soft drinks, but not appreciably so. The typical 32-ounce Powerade contains 280 calories. A 20-ounce bottle of Gatorade sets you back 150. Also, products such as Vitamin-Water and Smartwater would leave most consumers to believe they are getting water with vitamins. This isn't the case. These drinks are flavored with crystalline fructose, a type of sweetener that adds 150 calories per 20-ounce bottle, the same as sugar. That's a lot more calories than most people think they are getting with their water! Finally, the labeling on these products is often deceiving. If you quickly look at the calories in a bottle of VitaminWater, for instance, you may think it contains only 50 calories, unless you also look at the number of servings. There are 2½ servings in a typical bottle. Who drinks just half a bottle? Multiply the number of servings by the calories and you'll see that a bottle totals 125 calories, not 50.

If you consumed the same calories from food, you might eat less because your brain would sense those calories and reduce your appetite later in the day. The same doesn't seem to hold true for liquids. In a Purdue study, researchers fed volunteers 450 calories a day of soda or jelly beans. Both contain rapidly digested sugar, but the jelly bean eaters compensated for the excess by eating less throughout the day. The soda drinkers did not.

Why are liquids less satisfying than even the least satisfying foods? The problem probably starts in the mouth. Part of the satisfaction of eating stems from the act of chewing and of feeling food in your mouth. You don't chew liquids. They pass through your mouth quickly.

They spend little time in your stomach, too. Unlike solid food, which needs to be churned and puréed by the stomach before moving into the intestines, liquids spend so little time in the stomach that they do not weigh it down for a long enough period of time to trigger stretch receptors to signal the brain that the stomach is filling up. As a result, the hunger hormone ghrelin, released by the stomach when it's empty, remains elevated.

Then liquids pass quickly through your intestinal tract, too. They evade every calorie-detecting mechanism in your body. None of this matters if you've consumed water, which contains no calories. It matters greatly, however, if you consume highly caloric sugar-sweetened beverages. Most soft drinks run you about 100 calories per 8 ounces. That's the size of a measuring cup, and no one drinks just a cup. The typical "small" beverage is 16 ounces these days, and large drinks are double or triple that size. One caloric drink a day can add anywhere from 200 to 820 extra calories, enough to cause you to *gain* ½ to 2 pounds a week.

The 40-ounce Super Big Gulp, for example, totals 800 calories. That's the amount in a meal and a half for some people. Yet your brain thinks your stomach is empty. Those calories come in, but hunger hormones remain elevated, so you continue to eat as you normally would.

## Appetite Stimulators

Sweet beverages may do more than evade your body's detection system. They may actually increase appetite. Penn State research shows that consuming a sugar-sweetened beverage with a meal can trigger you to eat roughly 105 more calories with the meal, and that doesn't count the calories in your drink. The more you drink, the hungrier you get!

The sweeteners in these drinks cause a sharp rise in blood sugar and insulin that then drops, causing rebound hunger. Studies show that drinks with protein—such as milk—are not as hunger producing as drinks made from sugar, such as soft drinks and fruit juice. Sugar-sweetened beverages may increase thirst as well, or do little to reduce it. In a Johns Hopkins study, forty-two men consumed 8 or 16 ounces of lemonade or water

. . . . . . . . . . . . . . . . . . . . . . . . . . . . . . . . . . . . . . . . . . .

**Skinny Solution:** Have you heard that drinking lots of water can help you lose weight? You won't lose hundreds of pounds by guzzling lots of water, but drinking water just before and during meals can help you fill up on fewer calories. Water mixes with the food you eat, filling up and weighing down your stomach to induce fullness. Because it's calorie-free, it reduces the overall calorie density of your meal. If you'd like to try it, drink one full glass of water before each meal and another with meals.

during a meal. The sugar-sweetened lemonade did not reduce thirst, but the water did. Consider that many people interpret thirst as hunger and you can see how this can cause you to overeat.

Surprisingly, the intense sweetness of these beverages may also increase your appetite, even if it comes from an artificial sweetener. In a U.K. study of twenty women, artificially sweetened beverages increased appetite, especially in women who normally did not drink them. In another study, women who consumed artificially sweetened lemonade went on to consume more calories the following day, especially from carbohydrates, than women who consumed sugar-sweetened lemonade or water. As it turns out, sweetness without calories makes you crave other sweet flavors, causing you to go in search of cookies, cakes, and pastries.

These diet beverages may also trick your brain into thinking "sweet" equals calorie free. As a result, many people who switch from sugar-sweetened beverages to artificially flavored ones don't consume fewer calories. They consume more because their brains lose the ability to tell the difference between highly caloric sweet foods and zero-calorie sweet foods. Their brains equate all sweet flavors with zero calories, and, as a result, fail to reduce appetite when they consume, pies, cookies, and other caloric sweet treats.

The average person drinks 18 ounces—two full glasses—of soft drinks a day. That's an extra 225 daily calories that do not turn down appetite. In just one month, that can add up to a 2-pound weight gain. It adds up to 24 pounds in a year. It's no wonder that the odds of becoming obese increase 60 percent for each can or glass of sugar-sweetened beverage you consume.

## How to Do It

Cut back on all sources of liquid calories. That includes soft drinks, fruit juice, flavored coffee drinks, and sports drinks. Your goal is zero or near-zero consumption of liquid calories. In addition to soft drink and fruit juice consumption, pay attention to what you add to calorie-free beverages. Coffee and tea contain no calories, assuming you do not add sugar and milk or cream. Once you start adding such ingredients, the calories add up quickly. Consider that a large Starbucks Mocha Coconut Frappuccino with whipped cream totals 710 calories. Instead, try an iced Americano with a splash of skim milk.

Eliminating these beverages all at once can result in withdrawal symptoms such as headache and lethargy. This stems partly from caffeine withdrawal. You can ease some of this discomfort by consuming a noncaloric caffeinated beverage such as tea or coffee as you cut back on soft drinks. The headache and lethargy may also stem from "sugar addiction." If you try to give up soft drinks cold turkey but find that you feel out of sorts, use a step-down approach instead.

**Step 1:** Make a firm rule that you will never drink two sweetened beverages in a row. In other words, for every sweetened beverage you consume, you also must consume a glass of water.

**Step 2:** Cut back even more, reducing your consumption by half. If you normally have four sweetened beverages in a given day, drop down to two of them and drink two additional glasses of water.

**Step 3:** Drop down to one beverage and an additional glass of water.

Use the water to replace caloric liquids. However, you don't have to drive yourself crazy by trying to guzzle gallons of water. I've seen some diets that tell you to walk around with a gallon container and drink as much as you can. There's no reason to drink so much that you feel the stuff swishing in your stomach.

**Skinny Solution:** If you would like to try diet beverages, do so, but keep careful tabs on your hunger levels and cravings in a food journal. If, after the switch, you find yourself giving in to cravings for cookies and other sweets, take that as evidence that these drinks are triggering those cravings.

## Make It Happen

If you've struggled to give up soft drinks or coffee drinks, you may be sugar addicted. I treated one young woman recently who told me that she didn't feel well if she didn't have a six-pack of Coke on a given day. Whenever she tried to cut back, she felt disoriented. She understood why she should stop drinking the soda, but the physical addiction blocked her from putting this advice into practice.

I suggested that she substitute a small protein snack for each soda. The protein snacks served as temporary lifesavers, providing her body with

## The Skinny on . . . Why Meal-Replacement Shakes Fill You Up

Meal-replacement shakes are thick, which helps induce fullness for two reasons. Unlike soft drinks, the thickness causes you to drink meal-replacement beverages more slowly. They linger for a longer period of time in your mouth. They also linger for a longer period of time in your stomach, where they weigh it down and trigger stretch receptors to turn off production of the hunger hormone ghrelin. In contrast to the pure sugar in soft drinks, most meal-replacement beverages contain robust amounts of protein and fiber.

appetite-blunting nutrition at a time of day when she usually dosed herself with pure sugar. They kept her afloat, so she could withstand the withdrawal. She also used the step-down approach (described on page 108) to wean herself off the soda. By the time she had stopped drinking the six-pack, she had dropped 35 pounds, all by making one simple change.

In addition to having a small protein snack, you can also try the following advice.

**Flavor seltzer with a lemon or lime.** Seltzer gives you the mouthfeel of a carbonated drink without the calories, and the lemon or lime adds flavor without sweetness. You can also flavor it with some herbal tea, a squeeze of orange, or a very small splash of juice (less than 1 ounce).

**Water down your caloric drinks.** Do you miss drinking something sweet? Slowly diluting the sweet beverages you drink can stop sweet cravings in some people. Dilute sweetened beverages with water or club soda. Add as much ice to the glass as you can fit before pouring. Start with a half-and-half mixture. Then increase the water to three-fourths of the glass. Eventually, try to keep the sweetened part of the beverage to no more than 1 ounce.

**If you have a soft drink or juice, have it while sitting up at a table.** Surprisingly, research shows that the position of your body as you drink a beverage affects whether that beverage will fill you up. If you drink a beverage while lounging—say, on the couch in front of the TV—it will land in the lowest part of your stomach, where it is least likely to stimulate stretch receptors.

**Drink the smallest portion possible.** If you have a 32-ounce soda sitting in front of you, you will drink a 32-ounce soda. Most soft drinks, sports drinks, and other flavored beverages come in bottles that are 2½ times their serving size. Pour them into an 8-ounce glass and then put the original bottle out of sight.

# 9

# The Skinny Movement Makeover

We thought Cindy had reached her goal weight. She'd already lost 20 pounds and her weight was stable. "These are great results," I told her. "I'm very happy with your progress. I think this is the best you can do."

About a year later, she came in for a routine follow-up. She'd dropped another 30 pounds. I was stunned.

"Have you changed anything?" I asked.

"No, I can't think of anything," she said. "I'm still following the maintenance plan you suggested."

I continued to question her. No one drops 30 pounds without doing *something* differently. I wanted to know what Cindy's something was. I eventually learned that she had moved to the suburbs and now lived a mile from the train. Each morning she walked to the train station, boarded a train, and walked another mile from her stop in the city to her office. In the evening she did the same in reverse. It totaled four daily miles of walking.

If she had been walking these four miles on a treadmill, I would have worried about her ability to maintain this change, but walking to and from the train station was a part of her everyday lifestyle. I knew she could keep it up, and she has.

## Why It Works

Cindy added her four miles of walking at the absolute best time in her weight-loss journey—once she'd reached a plateau. I've seen many diets that recommend cutting calories once you hit a plateau. If you're not losing on 1,800 calories, these diets may tell you, drop down to 1,500 and then 1,200 calories. That's just crazy. You can't diet your way through a plateau.

When my renowned colleagues at Columbia, Dr. Michael Rosenbaum and Dr. Rudolph Leibel, studied the metabolic rates of people who had recently lost roughly 10 percent of their weight by dieting, they determined that this small weight loss slowed calorie burning significantly. All of the reduction occurred within their muscles during physical activity. Their muscles conserved calories during everyday tasks such as walking to and from the mailbox, the car, and the office. The net effect was a 42 percent reduction in the number of calories burned during movement! Whereas most people burn about 100 calories for every mile they walk, these dieters were burning only 58.

Why did their metabolisms slow so dramatically? Leptin. As I've mentioned, weight loss causes leptin levels to drop. When leptin is low, metabolism slows. With low leptin levels, the muscles of these dieters became more efficient, learning how to go farther on less fuel.

Sure, you can *try* to eat even less to work your way through such a plateau, but you'll only battle extreme hunger and your metabolism will slow even more. You repeatedly battle diminishing returns for your hard efforts.

It's much more realistic to exercise your way past a plateau. Once you start exercising, and, consequently, building muscle mass, you can further shrink your fat stores without experiencing another drop in leptin, finds research from the University of Las Palmas de Gran Canaria in Spain. In a study done at this institution, participants dropped 7 percent of their fat stores, but kept leptin levels steady with the help of a strength-training program. Regular exercise also helps sensitize the brain to leptin by driving down triglycerides, those blood fats I mentioned that may block leptin from reaching the fullness center. It also sensitizes muscle cells to insulin and brain cells to dopamine.

Every pound of muscle in your body burns 35 to 50 daily calories, even when it's not moving. Fit muscles also tend to lose calories as they produce heat, which is why exercise makes you feel hot. For these reasons, regular exercise blunts the improvement in muscle efficiency normally caused by weight loss, helping you get past weight-loss plateaus. Your body can't compensate for the change in efficiency brought on by exercise.

Additional reasons to move include the following:

**Better health:** Research shows that, even in the absence of weight loss, exercise reduces risk for many weight-related conditions, including heart disease and diabetes.

**Improved mood and well-being:** Regular exercise elevates mood, improves sleep, and reduces joint discomfort. Research shows that it's just as effective as antidepressants at lifting depression. People who

. . . . . . . . . . . . . . . . . . . . . . . . . . . . . . . . . . . . . . . . . . . . . .

## The Skinny on . . . Whether Exercise Makes You Hungry

Each time you exercise, you create a calorie deficit, and your brain may try to correct that deficit by increasing hunger. Most people, however, do not completely make up for burned calories when they eat. They feel somewhat hungrier in the hours after exercising, and they consume slightly bigger portions, but studies show that they remain in a slight calorie deficit for the rest of the day. In other words, they don't replace all of the calories that they burned.

Exercise tends to cause overwhelming hunger only in the following situations:

- You exercise very intensely for a long period of time (more than an hour). This can put you in a low-blood-sugar state that triggers excessive hunger.
- You exercise on an empty stomach. Again, blood sugar drops too low, causing an excessive appetite.
- You exercise in order to eat more. If during every mile you walk or run, you think about what you can now eat because of all of the calories you've "incinerated," you'll probably arrive home, head to the ice cream, and undo all of your hard work. Don't reward yourself for exercise by eating more. Just try to eat normally.

exercise regularly also report feeling more in control of their health and more satisfied with their social lives. All of these factors improve your quality of life, making you a happier, more energetic person, and more likely to stick with your healthy eating choices.

## Shouldn't I Exercise From the Beginning?

You can exercise from day one, but you don't *have* to. I believe in success, and after more than twenty years in this field, I know that the most successful people focus on changing their eating habits first and on exercise second. As I've mentioned, I'm a numbers guys and a research guy, and when it comes to exercise and weight loss, the numbers add up in favor of the food. Kelly Shaw, who works at the Department of Health and Human Services in Tasmania, Australia, analyzed forty-three diet- and exercise-related weight-loss interventions dating back to 1985. When she started the study, she thought she was going to prove what everyone suspected was true: that dieting without exercise results in weight regain. She didn't.

As Shaw discovered, six months of dieting without exercise allowed most people to drop an average of 20 pounds. Six months of exercise,

● ● ● ● ● ● ● ● ● ● ● ● ● ● ● ● ● ● ● ● ● ● ● ● ● ● ● ● ● ● ● ● ● ● ● ● ● ● ● ● ● ● ●

### The Skinny on . . . Why Your Exercise Machine Readout Isn't Accurate

Occasionally, one of my patients will tell me, "I burned nine hundred calories on the elliptical machine yesterday!" It sure sounds impressive, but I know the number is probably exaggerated. Many cardio machines don't calculate calorie burn effectively. What you burn during a workout is based on your body size, your gender, and your genetics. Most machines don't ask for this data, so their readouts are often based on an average person who could very well burn more calories during a given workout than you do. Plus, small changes in posture, such as pressing your hands against the rails as you walk, can dramatically reduce the calories you burn while using these machines. The machines can also lose their calibration, causing the readouts to be faulty.

without dieting? These folks lost just over 4 pounds. If you have the time and motivation to do only one or the other, changing the way you eat is clearly the more effective of the two strategies, at least in the beginning. Small dietary changes, such as the ones suggested in this program, can easily slice off up to 500 daily calories. You'd have to walk or run more than five miles to burn off that much, which is why nutrition easily wins when it comes to weight loss.

Don't get me wrong. Exercise is important for your health and your long-term weight maintenance. It's critically important for getting past a plateau, and for helping you reverse fullness resistance. It's required once you hit your first plateau.

## How to Do It

Food and Drug Administration guidelines recommend up to ninety minutes of daily exercise to lose weight. If you're sitting in your La-Z-Boy and thinking to yourself, "Yeah right, like I'm ever going to do that," I'm with you. I hear that all the time, and I have something to tell you that I think you're going to like to hear. Although that amount of exercise would undoubtedly help you drop pounds, it's not realistic and not necessary.

First, trying to exercise for this amount of time often backfires because it's not sustainable. Second, those guidelines were developed, in part, to allow people to lose weight through exercise alone. Well, as I've already mentioned, exercise just does not add up to a heck of a lot of lost pounds. Third, the ninety-minutes recommendation is based on the idea that the calories burned during an exercise session is the most important reason to exercise. Yet calorie burning is probably the least important reason to get moving, for a number of reasons.

- Charts that list how many calories you burn during a given exercise are wildly misleading because they don't account for the number of calories you would burn by doing nothing. For example, you may see a chart that claims that jogging burns 580 calories in an hour. Sure, that sounds like a lot, but you would normally burn 174 lying in bed, so your true calorie burn is 406.
- It takes a lot of exercise to burn a modest amount of calories. During intense exercise, you may burn 500 calories, an amount that is easily undone by eating just one Danish

pastry (which many people can consume in just a few minutes).

- The more familiar you are with an exercise, the fewer calories you will burn. As you get used to using an exercise bike or walking on a treadmill, for example, you may burn 10 percent fewer calories because of the familiarity effect. If you burned 200 calories when you were starting out, the same workout eventually burns just 180.
- As you lose weight, you'll burn fewer calories during exercise.
- Many people who focus on how many calories they burn also use the idea of those burned calories as a reason to reward themselves with food, which often backfires because it's all too easy to eat more calories than you burn.

I'd much rather you thought of exercise as a way to reverse fullness resistance, feel better, improve your mood, improve your metabolism, and improve your health. You can do all of this with just small amounts of daily movement, such as a ten-minute walk before meals, and a once or twice weekly strength-training program done at home. You need not go to the gym. You need not wear Spandex or sweats. You need not break a sweat.

My plan involves a two-step approach to exercise:

**Step 1—lifestyle movement:** You'll incorporate more movement into your everyday activities, such as taking the stairs and walking or riding a bike instead of driving. Once this daily movement becomes habitual, you'll increase the intensity by inserting periodic bursts of faster walking. This increase in intensity helps stabilize leptin levels.

**Step 2—strength training:** On pages 119–131 you'll find a progressive program you can do at home. It starts with just four exercises—for a total workout time of about ten minutes—and builds to nine exercises, for a total workout time of about twenty minutes. You'll do it once or twice a week, and it's so simple, you can do it in your pajamas.

Let's talk about how you'll accomplish Step 1. Make it your goal to walk roughly thirty minutes a day. I'm not talking about one thirty-minute walk, although that's great if you feel inclined. I'm talking about numerous five- to ten-minute walks, and I'm using the word *walk* liberally. Any movement counts, whether it's gardening, cleaning, or playing actively with your children or pets.

Study after study shows that short, periodic bursts of activity—such as house cleaning, gardening, and walking—can add up over time to a significant drop in weight. When done consistently, this unstructured "exercise" can be just as effective as going to the gym and sweating it out on a stair machine or treadmill for ninety minutes a day.

Most people spend eight or more hours in bed and half of their wakeful hours sitting. Reverse this. Stand up and walk whenever possible. Never drive in your car when you can walk or cycle. Use these easy ways to get moving:

- If you live in a small town or city where everyday conveniences such as the bank, restaurants, and other stores are close together, complete these errands on foot or on a bicycle.
- Never use a drive-through. Physically getting out of your car and walking into the bank or pharmacy does more than get you moving. It also brings you in contact with people, which, research shows, can lift your mood.
- If you live in a city, walk whenever you need to go less than ten or fifteen blocks.
- When you go to the mall, park at the first spot by the entrance to the lot rather than by the door. Walk the perimeter of the mall before allowing yourself to go inside a single store.
- Use the stairs instead of the elevator, or take the elevator to the floor below where you need to go and walk up one flight of stairs.
- Whenever you are early for an appointment or encounter a long wait, give the receptionist your cell phone number and take a walk while you wait. This will reduce your annoyance and help you slip in some extra walking.
- Play actively with your kids. Do Dance Dance Revolution with them. Hit a tennis ball, play catch, or run through a sprinkler. Get the Nintendo Wii Fit. It looks great.
- Walk before or after meals.

The more you put your mind to it, the more ways you'll find to move. Once you are firmly established with this walking habit, insert bursts of more intense activity. For example, as you walk, speed up your pace for one to two minutes, as if you were late for a meeting. Then slow down to your usual pace for a minute or two before speeding up again.

Now, let's talk about Step 2. Move on to Step 2 once you are walking for thirty or more daily minutes. Step 2 will strengthen your muscles, improve your metabolism, and help further reverse insulin resistance. If you take a look at the exercises I recommend on pages 119–131, you'll probably come to one conclusion: that program looks pretty easy. It's easy for a reason. I want you to do it and keep doing it.

Ideally you would strength train two to three times a week, doing multiple sets with fairly heavy weights. That type of program will build muscle in record time, but it's not realistic. You can still build muscle and improve your metabolism with this more moderate program. You just won't build as much muscle as with these more involved programs, but you'll be more likely to stick with it. The most effective strength-training program in the world is completely ineffective if you find it so boring and time consuming that you can't get yourself to do it.

Use these tips when starting and maintaining a strength-training program.

**Do it in the morning.** This is usually the best time of day for most people because it's the time of day that gives you the most control. You just set your alarm a few minutes earlier and get it done. If you wait until later in the day, you risk the chance of random life events (your kid has the flu and needs you to pick him up from school, your boss wants you to work late, your spouse wants you to run to a couple of stores on your way home from work, a friend calls with a life emergency) derailing your best exercise intentions. If you exercise in the morning, you'll feel good about your efforts all day long, which can help you stick to your healthy eating choices.

**Do it not long after eating.** If you exercise in the morning, have a light snack first. If you exercise later in the day, do it within an hour or two of eating. Otherwise you risk getting excessively hungry and undoing your good efforts by grabbing a doughnut afterward.

Skinny Mini: In New York, fitness centers know that people are not willing to travel more than twelve blocks to get to a gym, so they offer generous incentives to first-time clients who live farther away. The reasoning? They want you to pay the initiation fees, exercise for a month or two, and never show up again. If you prefer to exercise at a gym, choose the gym closest to your home, even if it doesn't have the flashiest equipment.

## Wall Push *Chest and upper body*

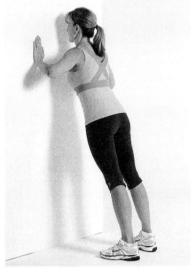 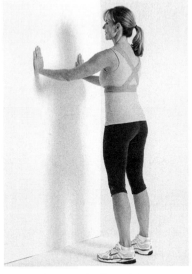

1. Stand with your elbows bent, your feet flat on the floor, and your palms against a wall slightly lower than shoulder height. Incline your body inward by walking your feet back.

2. Keeping your back straight, extend your arms as you push away from the wall. Return to the wall and repeat. Complete up to 20 repetitions.

## Standing Reciprocal Reach *Back, shoulders, and buttocks*

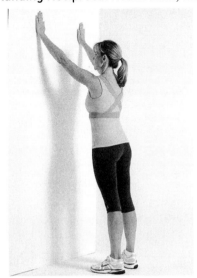

1. Stand facing a wall. Place your palms against the wall and extend your arms overhead. Step back 1½ to 2 feet, until your body is a flat plane and you feel the weight of your body against your hands and arms.

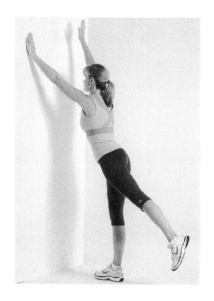

2. Raise your right arm and left leg as high as you can behind you. Hold for a count of 5. Lower and repeat with your left arm and right leg. Continue switching sides until you've completed up to 20 repetitions.

**Wall Sit** *Legs, buttocks, lower back, and abdomen*

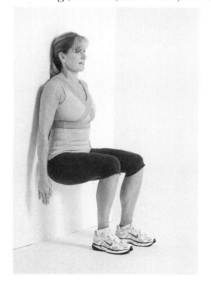

1. Stand with your back to a wall. Walk your feet forward as you bend your knees and slide your back down the wall until your legs are bent at right angles. Firm your abdomen and press your lower back into the wall. Hold up to 1 minute.

**Tummy Tuck** *Abdomen*

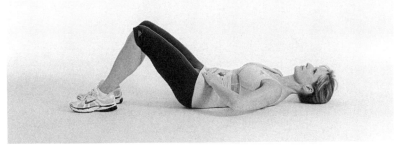

1. Lie on your back with your knees bent. Place your hands against your tummy. Exhale as you suck your tummy inward, as if you were trying to slip into a very snug pair of jeans. Hold for a count of 5; release and repeat up to 20 times.

## Intermediate Program

For this program, you will need a resistance band with handles, available online and at sporting goods stores. Start with the lightest band and work your way up to the highest resistance band over time.

**Knee Push** *Chest and arms*

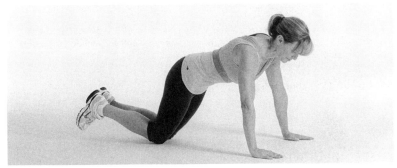

1. Kneel with your knees touching the floor, your palms under your chest, your back flat, and your elbows extended.

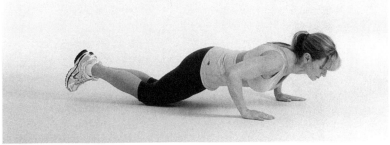

2. Slowly bend your elbows as you lower your chest toward the floor. When you are about 2 inches from the floor, rise back to the starting position. Repeat up to 15 times.

## Prone Reciprocal Reach *Back, shoulders, and buttocks*

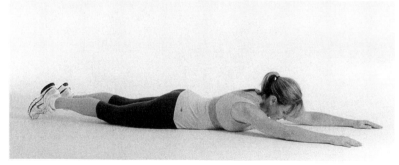

1. Lie on your tummy. Extend your arms overhead.

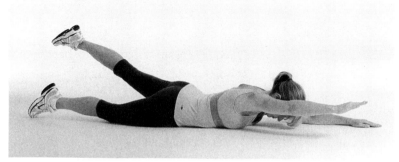

2. Lift your right arm and your left leg. Hold for a count of 5. Lower and repeat with your left arm and right leg. Continue to alternate sides until you've done up to 20 repetitions.

## Front Lunge *Legs and buttocks*

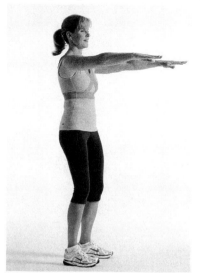

1. Stand with your feet under your hips. Extend your arms out in front at chest level for balance.

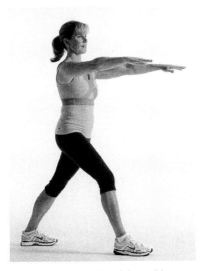

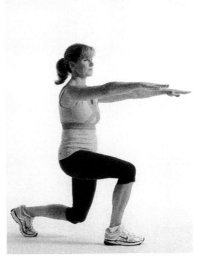

2. Step forward about 2 feet with your right leg. Bend your knees and drop down into a lunge.

3. Once both knees bend at right angles, rise and return to the starting position. Repeat with your left leg. Continue to alternate right and left until you've completed up to 20 repetitions.

## Butterfly with Exercise Band *Upper back*

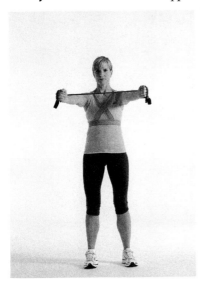

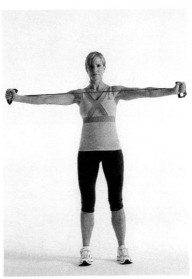

1. Stand. Wrap an exercise band around your hands. Extend your arms in front at shoulder height.

2. Pull the ends of the band, spreading your arms to the sides. Pinch your shoulder blades together as you stretch your arms. Hold 5 seconds, return to the start, and repeat up to 10 times.

## Biceps Curl with Exercise Band *Upper arms*

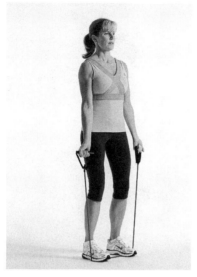 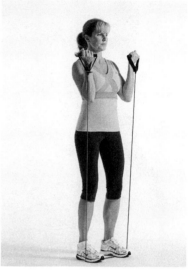

1. Stand on the middle of an exercise band, holding the ends in each hand, your hands extended down.

2. Keeping your wrists straight, bend your elbows, raising your hands toward your upper arms. Hold 5 seconds; release and repeat up to 20 times.

## Triceps Kickback with Exercise Band *Upper arms*

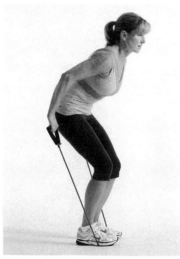 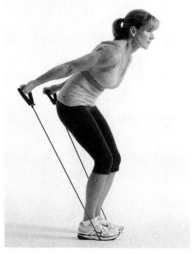

1. Stand on the middle of an exercise band, holding the ends in each hand, your hands extended down. Bend your knees slightly and bend forward from your hips, keeping your back flat.

2. Pull the band up and back. Hold for a count of 5; lower and repeat up to 20 times.

**Knee-Up** *Abdomen*

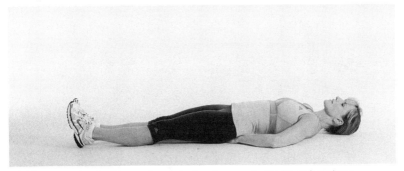

1. Lie on your back with your hands just under your buttocks, palms down.

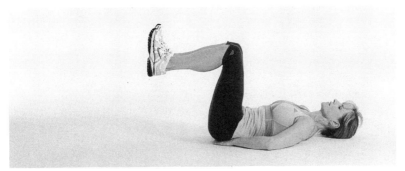

2. Slowly lift your knees into your chest, hold 5 seconds, and then extend your legs, just grazing the floor. Repeat up to 20 times.

## Advanced Program

Many of the advanced exercises require using dumbbells. Choose a weight light enough for you to lift without straining, but heavy enough so the last 2 or 3 repetitions feel challenging. For many people, 10- to 15-pound dumbbells work best for the overhead press, 5- to 10-pound dumbbells for triceps kickbacks, 10- to 20-pound dumbbells for biceps curls, and 15- to 20-pound dumbbells for lunges. As you gain strength, the exercise will eventually feel somewhat easy, even at the last repetition. At that time, increase your dumbbell weight.

## Overhead Press *Shoulders*

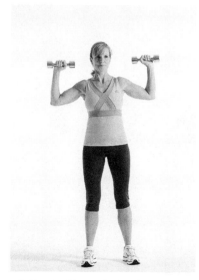 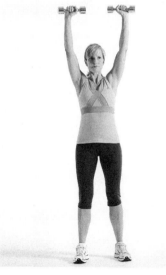

1. Stand with your feet under your hips and a dumbbell in each hand. Lift the dumbbells to shoulder height.

2. Extend your arms as you press the weights toward the ceiling. Lower and repeat up to 20 times.

## Triceps Kickback *Triceps*

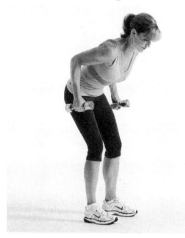 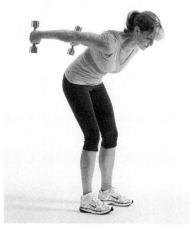

1. Bend your knees slightly. Grasp a dumbbell in each hand. Bend your elbows, holding the weights so that your upper arm is parallel to the floor and your forearm is perpendicular to the floor. Keep your upper arms as close to your torso as possible.

2. Extend your arms, lifting the weights behind you. Lower and repeat up to 20 times.

## Biceps Curl with Dumbbells *Upper arms*

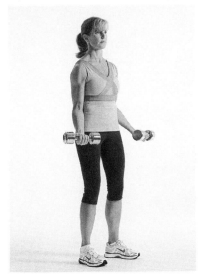 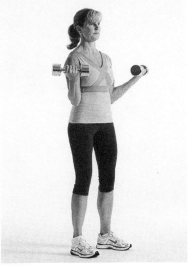

1. Stand with a pair of dumbbells in either hand, your hands extended down.

2. Keeping your wrists straight, bend your arms, bringing your hands toward your upper arms. Lower and repeat up to 20 times.

## Push-Up *Chest and arms*

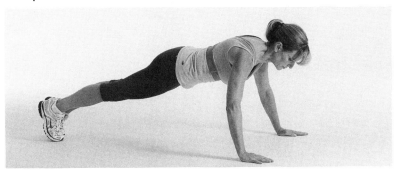

1. Come into a plank position, with your legs extended and your hands on the floor under your shoulders.

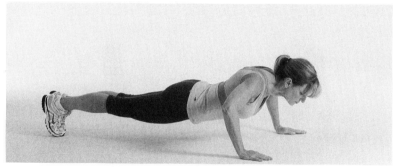

2. Slowly bend your elbows, bringing your chest toward the floor. When you get within 2 inches of the floor, push back to the starting position and repeat up to 15 times.

## Flat Cross Twist *Abdomen*

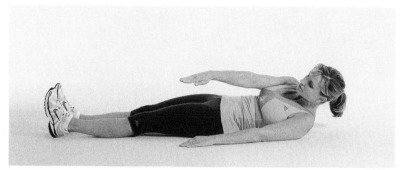

1. Lie on your back with your arms by your sides. Raise your right shoulder as you reach your hand toward your left knee. Lower and switch sides, alternating sides for a total of 10 to 15 reps.

## Crunches *Abdomen*

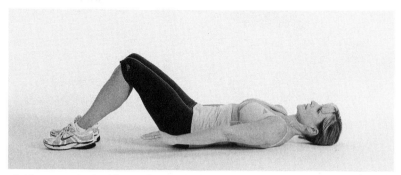

1. Lie on your back with your feet on the floor and your knees slightly bent. Rest your hands at your sides.

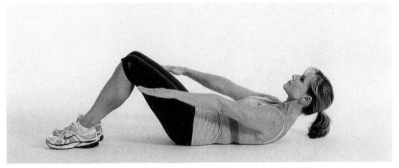

2. Raise your head and shoulders until your middle back lifts off the floor. Reach your hands toward your knees. Hold 3 seconds; lower and repeat up to 20 times.

## Lunge with Dumbbells *Legs and buttocks*

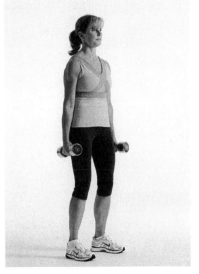

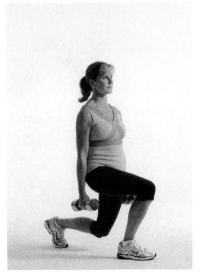

1. Stand with your feet under your hips. Grasp a pair of dumbbells in each hand.

2. Step forward about 2 feet with your right leg, bend your knees, and drop down into a lunge. Once both knees bend at right angles, rise and return to the starting position.

3. Repeat with your left leg. Continue to alternate right and left until you've completed up to 20 repetitions.

**Bridge with Ball** *Buttocks, legs, and back*

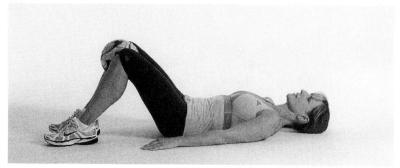

1. Lie on your back with your knees bent. Place a small ball (such as a children's ball or a soccer ball) between your knees. Rest your arms at your sides.

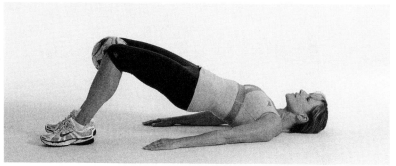

2. Press into your feet as you lift your buttocks, pressing your hips toward the ceiling. Hold for a count of 5; lower and repeat up to 20 times.

**Back Extension** *Lower back*

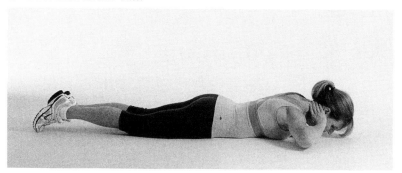

1. Lie on your tummy. Place your hands behind your head, elbows out to the sides. Extend your legs and tuck your tailbone.

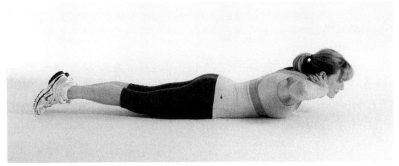

2. Lift your upper body as high as you can. Hold for a count of 5; lower and repeat up to 10 times.

## Make It Happen

Roughly half of people who start an exercise program stop within six months. I want you to stick with your new exercise habits for a lifetime. Use this advice:

**Don't do it for vanity.** Find a reason to exercise that has nothing to do with your body size or shape. Studies done at the University of Michigan show that women who work out just to get toned or to drop pounds tend to exercise about 40 percent less than women who exercise for other reasons, such as reducing stress, boosting mood, or maintaining a good social life (and yes, exercise really can do all of that, and more). So think about ways to move that you may find enjoyable. Do you like the outdoors? Then think about walking at a park once a day. Do you enjoy talking with friends? Consider meeting a friend each morning or evening for a social walk. Do you enjoy feeling a sense of accomplishment? Then set small goals and try to reach them.

**Wear a pedometer.** Pedometers are great motivators. Wear one for a few days to get a baseline. Most sedentary adults take about 5,000 steps a day. Try to double your number of daily steps.

**Think small and reward yourself often.** How confident do you feel about your ability to walk five minutes a day? How about ten? How about fifteen? There's no right answer here. It's better to start small, with an amount of exercise that feels comfortable and nonintimidating, and slowly add to that amount over time than it is to make a huge change that leads you to doubt your abilities to succeed. Each time you accomplish a small goal, you become more confident in your abilities, which helps you accomplish a larger exercise goal in the future. On the other hand, if you set lofty New Year's resolution–style goals and then continually fail to reach them, you continually erode your self-confidence.

Set the smallest goals possible—goals that you know, without a doubt, you can accomplish. Keep track of your exercise in your daily journal. Write down every small step in the right direction. Once a week, flip through your journal to see how far you've come. This will help you put the focus on your successes rather than your failures, helping to build your confidence.

**Don't worry about intensity until you've been exercising for a while.** Half of people who do vigorous exercise drop out, compared to 30 percent of people who do more moderate exercise. Any exercise—even at a very slow pace—is better than no exercise at all. If you hit a plateau, you can consider doing more intense exercise such as interval training, in which you vary the intensity of your activity, but do so only after you've established a firm exercise habit in the first place.

**Move daily rather than weekly.** I'd rather you did a little exercise every day rather than a lot just once or twice a week (or once a year on the second day in January). Daily exercise, even just small amounts of it, keeps muscle cells receptive to the hormone insulin. Just two days of in-activity, according to University of Missouri–Columbia research, causes insulin sensitivity to drop by one third. This means that insulin can't easily get sugar into muscle cells, so it puts it in fat cells, instead. More important, I've found that it's easier for most people to get into the habit of moving a little every day. It's a lot more intimidating to work out for sixty minutes, even if you are doing it just once a week, than to work out a little every day.

Skinny Mini: Participants in a University of Missouri–Columbia study who walked with a dog started with three ten-minute walks a week and naturally increased their time and duration to five twenty-minute walks a week. They also lost 14 pounds in a year.

**Pair movement with something you do every day.** If you get a structured break at work, go for a walk rather than standing by the watercooler or sitting in the break room (which is only going to tempt you to eat). Or do it just before or after meals.

**Investigate walking routes.** Research shows that people tend to walk longer and more often when they know the locations of a number of different parks, trails, neighborhoods with sidewalks, recreational facilities, and indoor malls.

**Line up an exercise buddy.** Walking with a partner will significantly increase the likelihood that you'll walk consistently. Not only does your partner make the walk more enjoyable, he or she keeps you accountable. It's easy to break a date with yourself, but harder to break a date with another person.

# Part Three

## Skinny Solutions

# 10

# The Solution for *Really* Stubborn Weight

You won't find this type of chapter in most diet books. That's because *most* diets are full of false promises. They want you to believe that dieting is easy, but it's not easy if you have an underlying problem that's working against your best efforts to change your eating and exercise habits. That's why I consider this chapter the most important one in this book. If you are following the *Skinny* menus and lifestyle tips in Part 2 and you have lost very little weight or continually battle extreme hunger, *something else is going on.* It's not you. It's your body.

Everyone I see in my practice at the Comprehensive Weight Control Program in New York has tried everything and can't lose weight. Some have even had weight-loss surgery, only to find that either they could not lose weight or they lost and then regained weight. I specialize in the "Intractable Patient." It's the title of a lecture I give at the Harvard obesity course, a continuing education course for physicians. Not every so-called intractable patient who sees me eventually loses weight, but I'm often able to help them succeed where others have failed by looking for simple, underlying problems such as prescription or over-the-counter medicines, a disease, or a stubborn weight-regulating mechanism. Use this chapter to troubleshoot the problem. Perhaps one of the following barriers stands in your way of success.

## Weight-Loss Barrier: Poor Sleep

Standing six feet tall, Stew was 60 years old and 295 pounds. His body mass index of 40 qualified him as a candidate for weight-loss surgery, but he wanted to lose the weight without going under the knife. His waist was 54 inches, his blood pressure 140/90, and his fasting blood sugar 110. He was taking more medicines than any reasonable person could ever keep track of, including four different medications to control his blood pressure, and they weren't working. I noticed that his eyes were bloodshot. He was also struggling to follow what I was saying. Occasionally I'd ask him a question and he'd stare into space, not realizing I was waiting for an answer.

I had a pretty good idea why he was struggling with his weight.

"How do you feel when you wake?" I asked.

"Tired," he said. "I need to sleep at least ten hours to feel rested."

His wife interrupted, "He snores. I sleep with earplugs."

I didn't need to hear more. I knew why Stew was struggling. He had sleep apnea, a condition that caused his airway to collapse as he slept, stopping his breathing hundreds of times throughout the night, repeatedly interrupting him from restorative sleep and either waking him or preventing him from getting the deep levels of sleep that he needed to feel rested. I recommended he get fitted with a device that blows heated, moist air into his airway, preventing it from collapsing. Stew started sleeping more soundly, and he started losing weight, too.

### The Skinny on How Sleep Affects Your Weight

Our bodies operate on a set clock, with certain processes taking place at night and others during the day. At night, the body secretes restorative hormones, lowers blood pressure, consolidates memories, and more. However, all of these restorative processes take place only if you sleep enough hours and at the right times. Sleeping fewer than seven hours or sleeping during the day rather than at night disrupts this clock for many people. Numerous studies show that as little as two nightly hours of sleep deprivation alters hormones that affect appetite. Levels of the fullness hormone leptin drop, and levels of the hunger hormone ghrelin and the stress hormone cortisol rise. Higher cortisol levels make cells more resistant to the hormone insulin, causing this fat storage hormone to rise, too. Two days of sleep deprivation resulted in a 24 percent jump in hunger and 23 percent rise in appetite for men who took part in a University of Chicago study. The men were particularly hungry for high-calorie sweets.

Sleep deprivation also makes you feel sluggish, so instead of walking across town, you take the bus. Instead of taking the stairs, you reach for the elevator button. Instead of gardening, you go straight to the hammock.

In the following pages, I've listed some of the more common reasons for sleep loss, along with what to do about them.

**Skinny Mini:** Researchers at the University of Bristol have followed the sleep habits and health outcomes of children, teens, and adults for many years and have arrived at some startling findings. Two-year-olds who did not get enough sleep were at a higher risk of becoming obese by age 7 than 2-year-olds who slept well. The researchers were able to show that lack of sleep disrupted fullness hormones, causing levels of hunger and stress hormones to rise and fullness hormones to fall. Over time, it led to insulin and leptin resistance.

## Advice For Sleep Apnea

People with sleep apnea snore loudly, often periodically choking or gasping for breath. When you progress into the deepest, most restorative levels of sleep, the muscles of the body become paralyzed. This prevents you from acting out your dreams and allows the body to rest and restore itself. The problem is that without the use of muscles, the airway easily collapses. The soft palate can relax and the tongue can fall back, blocking your airway.

Once the airway is blocked, breathing stops until brain oxygen levels drop enough to signal the brain that something is wrong. Then the brain pulls the body out of deep sleep, activating the muscles that control breathing, and you wake. Imagine how rested you would feel if someone shook you awake twenty times per hour, every hour, while you were

### Do You Have Sleep Apnea?

If you answer yes to any of the following questions, you may have sleep apnea:

Do you snore loudly, sometimes gasping for breath?
Do you feel tired when you wake in the morning?
Do you wake with a headache?
Do you feel tired during the day?
Do you tend to nod off while sitting, reading, watching television, or driving?
Do you have trouble concentrating or remembering things?
Are your eyes frequently bloodshot?
Do you wake frequently at night to urinate?

If you answered yes to one or more questions, discuss these symptoms with your doctor.

• • • • • • • • • • • • • • • • • • • • • • • • • • • • • • • • • • • • • • • • • • •

asleep. Just last week I saw a man who stopped breathing sixty-two times per hour! You may wake for such a brief period of time, however, that you don't remember waking at all. That's why so many of my patients are surprised when I suggest they have a sleep disorder such as sleep apnea because they tell me they're sleeping.

Sleep apnea is more common in men, people over age 40, and people with a wide neck circumference. As you gain weight, fat can build up around your airway, narrowing it and causing breathing problems. If your neck circumference is larger than 16 inches in women and 17 in men, you have a much greater risk of developing sleep apnea. This doesn't mean you are immune to sleep apnea if you are a young woman with a smaller neck circumference. I've treated patients who were young and only moderately overweight who had this sleep problem. They may have had a structural problem with their mouth and tongue.

**Don't drink alcohol or take sleeping medications.** Both relax the airway even more, making it more likely that it will collapse. I often ask my patients whether they've felt more fatigued the morning after taking sleep medicine. If the answer is yes, I consider investigating for apnea.

**Stay off your back.** Your soft palate and tongue fall back when you sleep on your back, increasing the likelihood that your airway will become blocked. Sleeping on your side or stomach alleviates apnea. Some people recommend sewing a tennis ball into a pouch in the back of a tight-fitting T-shirt and wearing it at night to encourage yourself to stay on your side.

**Ask your doctor about a sleep study and CPAP.** CPAP stands for *continuous positive airway pressure.* It is a mask that you wear over your nose during sleep. Air from an attached device comes through the mask and gently blows heated air into your nasal passages, preventing the throat from collapsing during sleep.

## Advice For Insomnia

Insomnia can cause you to toss and turn to get to sleep; wake you repeatedly at night; prevent you from entering the deepest, most restorative stages of sleep; or wake you too early in the morning. If you think you have insomnia, discuss the problem with your physician, and try the following remedies.

**Avoid caffeine.** Caffeine remains in your body anywhere from three to twelve hours, producing alertness. Slowly wean yourself off it by increasing your number of caffeine-free hours before bedtime and alternating each caffeinated beverage you consume with a decaffeinated beverage.

**Don't drink before bed.** An alcoholic drink may get you to sleep more quickly, but it may disrupt sleep later in the night, waking you repeatedly. It also prevents you from entering the deepest, most restorative stages of sleep.

**Don't eat too much before bed.** Besides being a good way to store calories efficiently and gain weight, eating just before bed can cause you to wake up in the middle of the night. Sometimes it's because you're burning the calories and that stimulates you to wake, and sometimes it's because you get heartburn, or reflux. Heartburn is a common cause of waking up at night. Taking antacids such as Zantac or Maalox can curb it.

**Take a bath before bed.** The water will warm up your core body temperature. Then as your body temperature drops, you'll get sleepy and more easily fall asleep.

**Exercise.** Regular exercise seems to improve sleep quality. For some people, exercising at night after dinner keeps them awake. If this happens to you, switch to a morning exercise routine.

**Sleep alone.** Many people wake less often if they sleep alone, away from the distractions of a spouse or pet.

### Advice for Sleep Skimping

Go to bed earlier, even if that means you need to get up earlier. If you are drowsy during the day, you are not getting enough sleep. What is keeping you up at night? When I ask my patients this question, I learn they are doing all sorts of things they don't really need to be doing. They are on the Internet. They are watching TV. They are doing laundry. Plan your day to allow yourself to go to bed earlier. Think about what you are doing at night that is keeping you up. Do you really need to be doing it?

### Advice for Shift Work

If you work at night or work a swing shift, you'll have a tougher time losing weight because you are working against your body's natural physiology. Your body will never adjust to shift work, but you can reduce its toll on your body and on your weight.

First, try to improve your sleep quality during the day by wearing earplugs and a sleep mask. Avoid large meals before your usual sleep time. And use the following advice:

**Exercise regularly.** Exercise may help shift your circadian clock, providing more rest during daytime sleep.

**Nap.** Talk to your supervisor about allowing a one-hour nap during the shift. A one-year study of twelve shift workers found that such a nap increased alertness during the shift by 44 percent.

**Wear sunglasses.** Block as much morning light as you can when you leave work, to continue to trick your brain into thinking that it's nighttime.

### Advice for Jet Lag

Flying through time zones forces the brain and body out of their natural sleep/wake pattern and into a new one. If you fly just once a year for vacation, this may not affect you, but if you fly frequently for business, jet lag may block your weight-loss efforts. Most people don't experience jet lag until they've crossed three or more time zones, and it generally takes one day to adjust to each zone you cross. Your body still wants to sleep at its usual time, so you toss and turn at your new bedtime. Then you feel tired and hungrier during the day.

If you will be at your destination for just a few days, stay on old time as much as possible. Eat meals based on your home time zone, exercise at your usual exercise time (old time) and sleep and wake according to this time (as much as your schedule allows). If you'll be staying longer, use this advice to encourage a faster transition to each new time zone:

**Get on new time as soon as possible.** Wake and sleep according to your new time zone, and eat meals according to it as well. This includes your plane flight.

**Walk outdoors whenever you feel tired during the day.** This will induce alertness.

**Get some sunlight.** If you are flying west, the best time to expose yourself to light is in the afternoon and early evening. If you are flying east, get outdoors during the morning and early afternoon. Exposure to light at these times of day will help reset your circadian clock to your new time zone.

**Eat a breakfast high in protein.** Protein will help induce alertness, so you can more easily stay awake when your body wants to sleep.

**Take a bath before bed.** A bath will warm up your core temperature. Then, as your body temperature drops, you'll feel sleepy.

## Weight-Loss Barrier: What's in Your Medicine Cabinet

Like so many of the people I counsel, Sarah seemed to be going about the business of weight loss in the right ways. She had managed to lose 100 pounds by following a low-carbohydrate diet and exercising thirty to ninety minutes a day. The problem was that she had regained 40 pounds in just four months, and she swore that she had not changed any of her lifestyle habits. "If anything, I'm eating less and exercising more than when I originally lost the weight," she told me. "What's going on?"

She was frustrated, and I didn't blame her. I was perplexed, too. We did a full panel of tests. Everything was normal. I asked her to keep a food journal, and sure enough, she was eating in a way that should have caused her to lose weight, not gain. I was stumped.

"Are you taking any medications?" I asked. "Perhaps something new?"

Bingo.

"I'm taking diphenhydramine to help me sleep," she said. "It's really noisy where I live, and the noise keeps me up if I don't take it."

Diphenhydramine is a potent antihistamine, and Sarah was taking three tablets a night, which is a big dose. We had found the cause of her problem. I switched her to a different sleep medication, and she started losing.

I've treated countless patients like Sarah, patients whose weight-loss efforts were blocked because they were taking certain types of medicines. In some cases their medicine had caused them to gain as much as 10 pounds a month when they had been diligently trying to *lose* weight.

Scores of medications have the unfortunate side effects of slowing your metabolism or increasing hunger. Medicines used to treat mood disorders, diabetes, and blood pressure are the most common culprits. If you've recently started a new medicine and have gained weight, ask your doctor whether weight gain is one of the side effects of that medicine.

**Skinny Mini:** Some of the following types of medicines may interfere with weight loss.

- Diabetes medicines
- Allergy medications
- Over-the-counter sleep medicines
- Medicines used to treat heart disease and high blood pressure
- Medicines used to treat depression and mood disorders
- Medicines used to treat epilepsy
- Medicines used to prevent migraine headaches
- Certain hormonal treatments for inflammation, fertility, and cancer

Work with your doctor to try to find an alternative that does not affect your weight. Do not stop taking any prescription medicine without consulting your doctor. Make an appointment with your doctor to discuss the possibility that your medicine is causing you to gain weight and to see if a better alternative is available.

You may need to try a few different medicines before you find one that works. I worked with a woman recently who was taking two weight-gaining medicines to treat her diabetes. Her physician had already tried to switch her to a weight-losing diabetes medicine, but she could not tolerate the other side effects. When she came to see me, she was demoralized because she thought she had run out of options. "There are three or four other medicines we could try," I told her. We tried another medicine, and she was finally able to lose weight—and control her diabetes.

# If You *Still* Can't Lose

This isn't going to make me popular, but it has to be said. Some people just can't easily lose weight. If you try everything in this book, get more sleep, and investigate your medicine cabinet and you *still* lose little to no weight, don't give up. You may not be able to lose weight, but you can hold steady and stop yourself from gaining. If you are 220 right now, that's better than 250, and 250 is better than 275. Hold the line.

Also consider talking with your doctor about using medicines and procedures that may help you lose, especially if your weight is affecting your health. Overweight and obesity raise risk for just about every single disease on the planet, including the top three most deadly ones: heart disease, diabetes, and cancer. You should not feel guilty if you can't lose weight with lifestyle approaches alone. That's like a heart disease patient feeling guilty for not being able to reverse the disease without medication or a cancer patient trying to cure cancer through exercise and diet.

To get your weight moving in the downward direction, you may need prescription help. So often people take medicines for all of the complications of their excess weight. Patients come to me already taking cholesterol-lowering medicines, blood pressure medicines, diabetes medicines, and the list goes on. The type of patient who sees me is typically on seven or more medications! Yet if they took a medicine that would help them lose weight, they might eventually be able to reverse these problems and many more. But doctors still don't prescribe medication for treating obesity as often as they should, considering the severity of the problem. One barrier is lack of insurance coverage, even though the weight loss achieved with medicine is about twice what you'd get with diet and exercise alone. The evidence is strong and growing that medication in conjunction with a program like mine can produce multiple health benefits.

Although just a handful of prescription medicines can help encourage weight loss and help with maintenance, many promising medications and medication combinations are now in development.

Because all medicines can have side effects, however, not everyone should take them. In general, I recommend that you consider weight-loss medicines only if your body mass index (BMI) is 30 or above, or if your BMI is 27 or above and you have a weight-related health complication such as high blood pressure, diabetes, or high cholesterol.

Talk to your health care provider about using one or more of the following weight-loss medicines.

## Meridia (Sibutramine)

**Background:** Meridia has been available in the United States for more than ten years. People who take the drug and lose weight usually experience side benefits that include reduced levels of triglycerides, LDL (bad) cholesterol, and total cholesterol. They also experience a boost in HDL (good) cholesterol.

**Dose:** 5, 10, or 15 milligrams in the morning.

**How it works:** It suppresses appetite and may have a modest metabolic effect.

**Potential benefit:** In studies, patients have lost an average of 10 pounds more than those who were taking a placebo and who were following a diet and exercise program. A long-term safety study is currently underway to determine whether Meridia is safe to use in higher-risk patients with health problems.

**Possible side effects:** Headaches, constipation, fatigue, and dry mouth. It may increase blood pressure and pulse in the short and long term, especially if weight is regained, so these need to be monitored every few months.

**Best for:** People who have a strong appetite, don't feel full after eating, think about food a lot of the time, are younger than age 35, and who don't have high blood pressure, heart disease, or cardiovascular risk factors.

## Allī (Orlistat)

**Background:** Formerly available by prescription under the name Xenical, this over-the-counter medicine has an excellent safety record. Allī contains half the dose of prescription Xenical. It has been shown to both improve weight loss and prevent weight regain. People who take the drug usually experience side benefits that include reduced levels of LDL (bad) cholesterol, blood pressure, and insulin levels. They also have improved glucose tolerance and levels of HDL (good) cholesterol.

**Dose:** 60 milligrams with each meal.

**How it works:** It decreases the absorption of fat in the intestine by about 25 percent. This reduces the amount of calories your body absorbs from the food you eat.

**Potential benefit:** Weight loss of about 50 percent more than you would lose with diet and exercise alone.

**Possible side effects:** Diarrhea, gas, bloating, and abdominal discomfort. A daily psyllium (fiber) supplement every evening may reduce these symptoms.

**Best for:** Allī is so safe that anyone with the BMI criteria described earlier can use it. It is most effective in people who gain weight despite not feeling hungry, have heart disease risk factors, eat out a lot, and are taking other medications.

## Adipex (Phentermine)

**Background:** Phentermine has been available in the United States for more than fifty years. It has been shown to help reduce weight by about 8 pounds more than diet and exercise alone. It is approved for three-month use. So far no long-term studies have been published showing that it is safe and produces health benefits, though at least one study is under way. Although this medicine is part of the phen-fen combination that was removed from the market many years ago, there is no evidence that taking phentermine alone results in heart problems. Phentermine is the most widely prescribed medication in the United States, but it's not available in Europe.

**Dose:** Usually half of one 37.5-milligram tablet in the morning.

**How it works:** It suppresses appetite and may have a modest metabolic effect.

**Potential benefit:** Weight loss of 8 pounds more than with diet and exercise alone.

**Possible side effects:** Headaches, constipation, fatigue, dry mouth, and anxiety. It may increase blood pressure and pulse in the short and long term, especially if weight is regained, so these need to be monitored every few months.

**Best for:** People who have a strong appetite, don't feel full after eating, think about food a lot of the time, are younger than age 35, and don't have high blood pressure, heart disease, or cardiovascular risk factors.

## Rimonabant (called *Acomplia* overseas)

**Background:** Rimonabant is the only prescription medication that turns down appetite by affecting the endocannabinoids system. Under the name Acomplia, it had been available in Europe since the middle of 2006. It is not available in the United States. Animal studies show that it reduces the consumption of fat and sugar.

**Dose:** 20 milligrams per day.

**How it works:** It reduces the overactivity of the endocannabinoid system in the brain, liver, muscle, fat cells, and pancreas. They reduce appetite and cravings for sweet, fatty foods, reduce the production of fat by the liver, and improve insulin sensitivity.

**Potential benefit:** In studies, patients lost 5 percent more weight when they took Rimonabant compared to diet alone. They lost more than 10 percent of their weight (an average of 23 pounds) when they used this medicine in conjunction with a program of diet and lifestyle change, and they maintained their weight loss for as long as two years (the length of the study). More important, the medicine also reduced blood sugar, triglycerides, and blood pressure, and raised HDL (good) cholesterol. In one study, it appeared to slow the progression of atherosclerosis, or coronary disease, and reduced the risk of death, but more research is needed to prove that the benefits outweigh the risks.

**Possible side effects:** Some study participants experienced nausea, depression, and anxiety.

**Best for:** People who have no history of depression, anxiety, or other mood problems; these medicines are contraindicated in those conditions. Rimonabant has been shown to be beneficial in people with cardiovascular disease and diabetes over and above its effect on weight loss.

## Medicines for Other Disorders

Although only a few FDA-approved drugs are specifically designed to induce weight loss, many other medicines that are approved to treat other health conditions—such as diabetes, migraines, and depression—can help. The following medications are good alternatives if you are currently taking a medicine that causes weight gain.

### Glucophage (Metformin)

**Background:** Designed to help people with diabetes control blood sugar, metformin may help reverse fullness resistance by suppressing the production of sugar by the liver and indirectly making cells more sensitive to the effects of the hormone insulin. By making cells more sensitive to insulin, metformin lowers insulin levels, which, in turn, helps lower cholesterol and triglycerides and also makes the brain more sensitive to the hormone leptin.

**Possible side effects:** In rare cases, metformin can cause a life-threatening condition called lactic acidosis, but usually only in people who have congestive heart failure. It may also cause headache, nausea, muscle aches, gas, and stomach upset.

**Best for:** People with type 2 diabetes, pre-diabetes, polycystic ovarian syndrome, or insulin resistance.

### Byetta (Exenatide)

**Background:** Byetta, an injectable medicine, helps enhance the secretion of insulin, helping to control blood sugar. In studies, it has been shown to enhance weight loss, inducing a 22- to 26-pound loss over eighty-two weeks, possibly by lowering appetite.

**Possible side effects:** Nausea, dizziness, diarrhea, low blood sugar, and allergic reactions.

**Best for:** People with type 2 diabetes that does not respond to other diabetes medicines such as metformin.

### Symlin Pen (Pramlintide)

**Background:** Symlin, an injectable medicine, mimics the hormone amylin, which helps control blood sugar levels. It also slows digestion. In research done by the company that makes it, study participants who injected it before meals lost an average of 8 pounds and reported decreased appetite. It may be even more effective in conjunction with other medications.

**Possible side effects:** Dizziness, nausea, and headache.

**Best for:** People taking insulin therapy. This medicine is used as a substitute for insulin, helping with weight loss.

### Topamax (Topiramate)

**Background:** Topamax is used to treat epilepsy and to prevent migraine headaches. One "side effect" is that it tends to reduce appetite and induce weight loss of about 13 pounds in overweight people.

**Possible side effects:** Cognitive problems, fatigue, abdominal discomfort, anxiety, dizziness, poor concentration, and mood problems.

**Best for:** People who have frequent headaches but gain weight on other commonly prescribed preventive migraine medicines.

## Wellbutrin (Bupropion)

**Background:** Used to treat depression and help people quit smoking, Wellbutrin helped women in a Duke University study lose more weight than a control group of women who reduced calories but did not take the drug. The average weight loss is about 6 pounds, but because many antidepressants cause weight gain, Wellbutrin can be very helpful.

**Possible side effects:** Dry mouth, headache, increased blood pressure, and seizures (rare).

**Best for:** People with depression who gain weight on other commonly prescribed medicines.

## What Not to Take

With effective and safe prescription and over-the-counter options, it's amazing to me how many people opt for supplements with no proven benefit. Please don't misunderstand me. I have no objection to alternative medicine. I'd be thrilled if any of these supplements were proven to actually work. The problem is that they haven't, and some may even be harmful.

The companies that sell them trick consumers with deceptive advertising. The FDA recently fined four companies $25 million for these false claims. To help you sort fact from fiction, I've listed what's known about some common weight-loss supplements.

## Hoodia

Despite claims that Hoodia is a "proven" weight-loss aid, no credible studies show that this supplement works to reduce body weight or yield a health benefit. This could be because it doesn't work, or because there isn't really any Hoodia, a rare ingredient, in the product, but we don't know because these products haven't been tested properly.

### Bitter Orange

Remember ephedra? It was so dangerous that the FDA, which generally does not regulate supplements, ordered it off the market. Bitter orange is the new ephedra, and it may be just as dangerous. Bitter orange contains the chemicals synephrine and octopamine, which are similar to the ingredient ephedrine in ephedra. These chemicals may cause high blood pressure and heart rhythm problems. Bitter orange can also interfere with other prescription medications you may be taking.

### "Cortisol-Lowering" Products

Once again, there is no credible evidence that these products work. Do yourself a favor, and don't fall for it.

## When to Consider Surgery

Some people who can't lose weight with lifestyle approaches or with prescription medicines opt for surgery as a last resort. Consider surgery if:

- Your BMI is 40 or higher.
- Your BMI is 35 or higher and you have a health condition such as high blood pressure or high blood cholesterol.
- You've tried the recommendations outlined in this book and can't make progress.

Obese people with health problems periodically ask me if they should try surgery first and skip the lifestyle approach. I answer yes only if they are at risk of dying in the immediate future because of their weight. This is extremely rare. Most people can lose weight and dramatically improve their health without surgery. Then if they end up going for surgery, they can honestly say they've done everything. Surgery for obesity presents the perfect example of risk vs. reward. The greater the risk, the greater the potential benefit in pounds lost.

One patient summed up the risk of surgery as follows: "I know surgery will reduce my risk of dying and help me to live a healthier, more enjoyable life, but if I die from surgery I'm gonna die a lot sooner."

If you decide to undergo surgery, know that in the right hands it's safer than many people think. It's true that all surgery poses a risk; you can die from any surgical procedure, including an appendectomy. Yet research shows that the 0.3 to 1.9 percent death rate associated with obesity surgery pales in comparison to the risk of death if you *don't* have surgery. If your BMI is 40 or higher, your risk of death if you *don't* lose weight is 6.17 percent during the next five years. In fact, a study done at the University of Utah School of Medicine determined that weight-loss surgery reduced the risk of death by more than 30 percent.

To reduce the risks associated with obesity surgery, choose a busy center and surgeon. The more often a physician and center do a surgery, the better they get at it. The Surgical Review Corporation (http://www.surgicalreview.org) and the American College of Surgeons accredit bariatric surgery programs. You can find a list of accredited programs at http://www.facs.org/cqi/bscn/index.html. Centers that are accredited not only must have a high enough volume of procedures to maintain proficiency, but their results are monitored to ensure that they deliver quality care.

Although many procedures can be performed to produce weight loss, two types of surgery are being done in 90 percent of patients.

## Lap Band

**What it is:** A surgeon places a silicone ring around the stomach, near the esophagus, creating a very small opening that only allows a small amount of food to pass at a time. This reduces the stomach's usual capacity to 5 percent, making it the size of an egg. On average, people who undergo lap band surgery lose 20 percent of their weight over time. The "lap band" name stems from the laparoscopic keyhole surgical technique used to insert the band.

**Pros:** The band is adjustable, so the surgery can be reversed by loosening the band if needed. The surgery is safer than gastric bypass because it is simpler.

**Cons:** This technique does not completely eliminate the desire to eat, allowing some people to override its effect. In our experience, some patients need to use medication in addition to the band to achieve best results.

**Best for:** Younger patients, people who need to lose lesser amounts of weight, and women who are planning to get pregnant.

### Gastric Bypass

**What it is:** Gastric bypass surgery permanently makes the stomach smaller, reducing it to about the size of an egg. The small pouch that is left is attached to a part of the intestine that is two feet down from the usual spot. It both reduces the amount of food you feel comfortable eating and very slightly reduces the amount of calories that are absorbed from the food you do eat. Most important, it prevents food from getting to the part of the intestine called the duodenum. This is the key difference between the gastric bypass and the lap band. When food bypasses the duodenum, a dramatic improvement in insulin sensitivity and blood sugar results, which can cure diabetes in more than 80 percent of patients.

**Pros:** This procedure usually yields more predictable and dramatic weight loss than the lap band. People lose an average of 33 percent of their weight. The desire to eat is reduced more than with the lap band as well. It is also performed through laparoscopic keyhole techniques.

**Cons:** The surgery is more invasive, with a more lengthy recovery time. It can also result in complications such as nausea, vomiting, vitamin or mineral deficiencies, ulcers, internal hernias, and a problem called *dumping syndrome,* in which too much sugar is "dumped" into your intestine at once, causing nausea, light-headedness, and diarrhea. Patients who have this surgery must take a lifelong regimen of vitamins. Perhaps because the egg-sized pouch stretches back to its former capacity, some weight can be regained.

**Best for:** Heavier patients, especially those who have diabetes.

## On the Horizon

The following procedures and techniques may soon be available.

### Sleeve Gastrectomy

In this procedure, part of the stomach is removed, molding the remaining portion into the shape of a thin tube, like a banana. The part of the stomach that is removed is a key source of ghrelin, the hunger hormone. Without this part of the stomach, less ghrelin is produced, reducing hunger levels. The shape of the stomach also restricts eating. Although available, this surgery is still considered experimental. Weight loss is about

25 percent in studies. Nutritional deficiencies are minor compared to gastric bypass.

## Endoluminal Surgery

Eventually, surgeons will be able to perform stomach surgery through the mouth, creating no incisions. Some physicians are already using this type of surgical technique to tighten gastric bands that have loosened over time. In one procedure, the endoluminal sleeve, a flexible tube is inserted through the mouth and into the duodenum to prevent the absorption of calories over just two feet of intestine. This technique is currently being studied, and preliminary results are very promising. The device is removable.

## Implanted Stimulators

This half-dollar-sized battery-powered device is implanted on the wall of the abdomen, where its electrodes attach to the wall of the stomach itself and emit impulses—much like a heart pacemaker—creating an exaggerated feeling of fullness when you eat. The operation to implant the device takes about one hour. Another stimulator targets the vagus nerve and is intended to block signals carried on the vagus nerve between the brain and the digestive system that control sensations of hunger, satisfaction, and fullness. It may also be turned off and is designed to be reversible, programmable, and noninvasively adjustable.

# 11

# The Solution For Lasting Weight Loss

Some surveys indicate that roughly 80 percent of people who lose weight regain most or all of it within a year. I want you to fall into the other category, the category of people we rarely hear about. I want you to be a part of the 20 percent who keep it off. To stay successful, use this plan for maintaining your weight loss.

Your first step in achieving lasting weight loss lies in determining when to stop losing and start maintaining. Many dieters pick an arbitrary finish line. They want to get down to a specific clothing size or see a specific number on the scale, but you just can't bully your body into losing the perfect amount of weight. Will you shed enough fat to fit into a size four, six, or eight, or into the jeans you wore in high school? I can't make that promise. At some point, as you lose weight, your body will fight back. It will defend your weight, and if you try to battle your body at this point, you'll end up feeling extremely hungry—despite choosing the most filling foods—and plateau anyway because your metabolism will slow. Trying to fight against this biology is like trying to push a car uphill. You may manage to go a few steps, but, eventually, biology wins, and your weight—like that car—goes in the other direction.

I know this isn't what you want to hear, and I wish I could tell you the magical secret that would allow you to get your body to that predetermined perfect place, but I just can't. I'd much rather be honest, and I'd much rather give you the tools to help you get to a healthy weight and then stay there. If you have a lot of weight to lose and can't consider some of the options such as medication and surgery discussed in chapter 10, I'd rather you lost a little weight and kept it off than lost a lot of weight and then gained a lot of it right back.

For this reason, I'd like you to forget about any preconceived notions you once had about your maintenance weight. Forget about that coveted number or clothing size. Instead, focus on your behavior—on successfully following this book's nutrition and lifestyle principles—and let your maintenance weight find you. To do so, follow the Phase 1 menus and exercise as directed in Part 2 for as long as you can. Once you feel deprived or bored with the Phase 1 choices, slowly transition to Phase 2 eating as described in chapter 3. Increase exercise as directed in chapter 9. Eventually, no matter how closely you monitor your eating or how diligently you exercise, you'll stop losing weight. This is your maintenance weight.

## Expect to Gain *a Little* Back

I've got some more news that you probably won't like. Most people gain back about 10 percent of their total weight loss. In other words, if you lost 20 pounds, you can expect to regain 2 to 3 pounds. If you lost 100, you may regain 10. Although few if any diet authors will admit it, *everyone* who loses weight regains a little. It's normal and it happens to almost everyone no matter how closely they follow their dietary and fitness regimens.

Why does it happen? You've transformed your body from one with chronically high levels of the fullness hormone leptin and low levels of the hunger hormone ghrelin to the opposite. Now leptin is low and ghrelin is high. These low leptin levels are, in part, what caused your plateau. As leptin levels drop, so does thyroid hormone, reducing metabolism so you burn fewer calories. Low leptin levels also allow hunger hormones to enter the brain unchecked.

We don't yet know all of the physical reasons why this happens, but regaining just a few pounds seems to increase leptin levels above some threshold level we haven't been able to identify, and brain chemicals stop sending out so many "eat more" and "burn less" signals. Your appetite and your metabolism reach a "truce," and your weight plateaus. Your body reaches an equilibrium that it can maintain.

## *Skinny* Secrets For Staying Skinny

To maintain your weight loss after you gain that initial 10 percent, do the following.

**Keep moving.** Continually look for ways to add more lifestyle walking to your daily repertoire. It's the best way I know of for overcoming plateaus and for maintaining weight loss. It's one of the few strategies that seem to help prevent low leptin levels from making your muscles more efficient. As a result, your metabolism can no longer act as such a brake on your weight loss. Some of my patients have plateaued, started a regular exercise program, and then experienced a new onset of weight loss to a lower plateau.

Exercise also helps overcome occasional overeating. Whenever you overdo it, your body has to decide what to do with the extra calories. If your muscles are "metabolically active" from exercising, calories will be sent to your muscles to be burned rather than to your fat cells to be stored. When researchers from Brown University and the University of Colorado studied longtime weight maintainers, they discovered that people who tended to regain weight got lax on their exercise habits. Those who kept the weight off tended to increase exercise as they maintained, with the average maintainer moving for sixty minutes a day, mostly through walking and light-intensity activities such as housework and gardening.

**Weigh yourself regularly.** Researchers from Cornell University asked a group of freshmen women to weigh themselves daily. They asked another group of women to weigh themselves just twice—at the beginning of the semester and at the end. At the end of the semester, the women who weighed daily gained no weight, whereas the women who didn't weigh gained between 4 and 8 pounds.

Why did daily weighing help? Even though the researchers provided the students with no information about dietary and exercise habits, the women who stepped on the scale each day naturally found ways to control their weight. If they saw an increase, they either ate less or moved more. They skipped snacks, skipped dessert, shrank portions, or stepped up their exercise efforts. They didn't count calories, but the feedback of the scale gave them constant nudges in the right direction.

You'll need to strike a careful balance between denial (*it's just water weight, I don't need to do anything differently*) and negativity (*I gained weight, I may as well eat whatever I want*). Many factors affect your weight beyond the size of your fat cells. You can expect your weight to fluctuate by about 5 pounds based on the amount of fluid your body is retaining, the regularity or irregularity of your bowel habits, and the amount of carbohy-

. . . . . . . . . . . . . . . . . . . . . . . . . . . . . . . . . . . . . . . . . . . . .

## Your Maintenance Graph

As you maintain, plot your gains and losses on a graph such as this one. Expect your weight to go up and down by a few pounds over and over again, but take corrective action if you end up connecting the dots and creating a line that continues to slant upward.

| Weight Gain or Loss | Days of the Month 1 2 3 4 5 6 7 8 9 10 11 12 13 14 15 16 17 18 19 20 21 22 23 24 25 26 27 28 29 30 31 |
|---|---|
| +5 | |
| +4 | |
| +3 | |
| +2 | |
| +1 | |
| 0 (maintenance weight) | |
| −1 | |
| −2 | |
| −3 | |
| −4 | |

drate stored in your liver and muscles. In the study I just mentioned, the college freshmen plotted their weight on a graph such as the one on page 158. A slight up-and-down line was nothing to worry about. A steady upward line, however, meant they needed to take corrective action.

What types of corrective actions should you take? Your first action should be to see if you've strayed from your Phase 2 menus or cut back on exercise. If so, reestablish those habits. If you're gaining despite carefully following the *Skinny* menus and tips described in the rest of this chapter, then see your doctor. You may have a health problem that's affecting your weight. Read chapter 10 to see if a sleep problem, a weight-gaining medication, or something else is affecting your weight. And try to make small dietary or lifestyle changes. Can you add five or ten additional minutes of movement a day? Can you fill up on fewer calories by eating even leaner, sneaking more veggies into a meat dish, or shrinking your starch portions?

**Fight hunger with lean protein plus vegetables.** As you maintain, you may find that at times, you feel hungrier than usual. During these times, increase your lean protein and your vegetable portions. By eating more of the right foods, you'll be able to more easily eat less of the wrong foods, and you'll more easily maintain your weight, too. But remember, just cutting back on calories is often not productive and can lead to overwhelming hunger because the counterbalancing systems get activated. To maintain your weight, it's always better to add than to subtract. Eat more filling foods, so they naturally displace the fattening ones.

**Turn off the tube.** People who regain weight tend to watch more TV than people who don't. The average American watches four hours a day, and more than 60 percent of average Americans are overweight or obese. Research completed at Brown University and a number of other institutions, however, shows that successful weight maintainers watch far less. More than a third of people who have maintained a 30-pound weight loss for a year or longer watch fewer than five hours a week and another third fewer than ten hours. The more TV study participants watched, the less they exercised and the more weight they regained.

**Be vigilant when life gets more stressful.** When patients come to see me after regaining weight, I always ask, "What changed?" Inevitably, something has. They take on more responsibility at work, move, have a baby, have a sick family member, or twist an ankle and can't walk as much. Whenever something changes in your life, it's time to be more vigilant. That's when you're most likely to backslide.

**Be consistent.** Use *The Skinny* to guide your eating during the week, on the weekends, and during vacations and holidays. Don't use it on some days and not on others. For example, many dieters like to have cheat days and cheat meals. They follow an eating approach flawlessly during the week and then go hog wild on weekends. That may be okay for some people, but this type of eating could damage your fuel gauge, causing you to start each week feeling excessively hungry from your weekend dessert-and-starch binge. Research shows that the most successful maintainers eat consistently every day, no matter the occasion.

In particular, *always:*

- **Eat protein for breakfast.** Although some people can get away with cereals, oatmeal, toast, juice, or another starchy breakfast once or twice a week, most maintainers can't eat these foods every day without noticing an increase in hunger. *Most* maintainers find that they must consume protein foods (from their Phase 1 breakfast options) most days of the week. The protein controls hunger and cravings for the rest of the day, so they naturally eat less for lunch and dinner. If you feel you have to have a starch for breakfast, have it with protein. For example, have a whole-grain English muffin with peanut butter, an egg, or turkey sausage.

- **Eat starch and dessert last.** Always consume starch or dessert at the end of the meal, after you've consumed your vegetables, salad, soup, and lean protein. This is when you'll have most control, so one reasonable serving of pasta does not turn into one gargantuan serving. For the same reason, never consume alcohol as an appetizer or just before your meal. Always have it with the main course or after dinner.

- **Use the three-bites rule.** I'm a weight-loss doctor. Does that mean I never eat cake or cookies? No way. As long as most of what you eat is rich in lean protein, fiber, and nutrients, you can occasionally eat sweets in moderation. The two important keys here are *occasionally* and *in moderation.* A few bites of dessert once or twice a week is probably okay for most people. A large serving every day probably isn't. Once you fix your fullness resistance, you can eat the small serving.

  When you have dessert, hold yourself to three or four bites, or about 100 calories. Most desserts served at restaurants contain 400 to 500 calories, or even more. This excess sugar and fat causes long-lasting rebound hunger. You'll find that you wake feeling hungrier the day after eating a huge dessert, and feel hungrier for a few days. Is that amount of hunger worth a huge piece of cake, pie, or cheesecake? It's not for me. Split desserts with two or three dining companions, and try to hold yourself to just a few bites. Pay careful attention to how the dessert tastes. You'll probably find that the first bite tastes the best, with each progressive bite tasting less intense than the first. By the fourth bite, the flavor has probably declined substantially. Once that happens, stop eating. If you keep on eating past that point, you may lose your sense of fullness and feel that you have to eat the whole piece, or another. Sound familiar?

- **Keep protein lean.** This allows you to eat a greater volume of food, so you fill up on fewer calories. Research on successful maintainers shows that most consume about half as much fat as the general population. Hold red meat to two to three times a week, opting mostly for skinless poultry or fish on the other days of the week.

## End the Yo-Yo Cycle

Have you ever wondered what causes yo-yo dieting, the phenomenon in which people get to their lowest weight and then regain everything right back? I can explain it to you. It involves two parts, one physical and the other psychological. First, your body resists weight loss because of changes I described earlier. Then you regain a few pounds to get your leptin levels back in equilibrium and you're a little nervous. Then you eat a big dessert, step on the scale the next day, see that you've gained weight, and get demoralized. Now you're hungry every day because fullness resistance is back. You feel as if nothing you try works, and you've stopped finding the point of trying so hard. So you give up.

To stop the yo-yo cycle, you first must understand and expect it. No matter how dedicated you are when you start maintaining, you'll eventually eat more than just a few bites of dessert. Everyone does. Expect that you will do this, so you can prepare yourself for the aftermath. You'll most likely do it on a holiday or at a birthday party. I've heard this story probably a hundred times. You're going to a birthday party and you want to eat some cake. You hardly eat anything all day long, banking your calories for the cake. You eat the biggest slice of cake that you can find, and perhaps a second slice as well. The sugar and starch in the cake spikes your blood sugar and insulin. With insulin this high, the brain wants to store these cake calories quickly, so a lot of the sugar goes straight to your liver, where it gets stored along with a generous amount of water. The liver converts some of it into fat, which settles in your fat cells.

You wake the next morning with a food hangover. It's very real, just like a hangover from alcohol. You're thirsty, because your body needs water to store the excess sugar. You're tired, hungry, and fuzzy-headed because the excessive release of insulin and other hormones has driven you into a low-blood-sugar state. The fastest way to feel better? Some hair of the dog, which is why you're craving sugar in the form of a breakfast pastry, a soft drink, juice, or a doughnut. Have those choices, however, and things will only get worse.

This is where you must stop the cycle. Don't reach for the doughnut. Don't have the soft drink. Don't berate yourself. Don't get demoralized. Instead, do the following.

**Get on the scale.** Doing so will help you recommit, but don't pay too much attention to the actual number. It's wildly exaggerated. I don't care how much overeating was involved. Even if you ate an entire cake along with a gallon of soda, it's physically impossible to gain 5 pounds of fat overnight. Each pound of fat adds up to more than 4,000 calories. You may have gained a fraction of a pound of fat, but you certainly did not gain 5.

Most of that 5-pound gain is from extra glycogen and water. You've gained liver weight, not fat weight. Your liver is the first reserve gas tank for your body. Whenever you overeat, your body stores most of the excess here, along with a lot of water. If you recommit to *The Skinny,* most of this liver weight will be gone within a few days.

The problem is that most people don't know this. So when they get on the scale and see the 5 extra pounds, they have a series of thoughts that do little to keep them motivated. They think things like "I really screwed up," "Now look what I've done," and "I worked so hard to get it off. How can it come back so quickly?" They are plagued with self-doubt. They question their judgment. They question their willpower. They question whether they have what it takes to keep the weight off.

You have what it takes. You won't gain anything if you recommit *right now.* It bears repeating: this is not fat weight. It's liver weight. If you get back on track now, it'll be gone in a few days.

**Be prepared for withdrawal symptoms.** You're going to feel as crummy as you did when you first started *The Skinny.* You're going to go through withdrawal, and this withdrawal will last longer because your hunger hormones will not drop as quickly now that you've reduced your body size. It may take as long as a week for you to completely recover.

**Eat more protein for breakfast.** Keep a meal-replacement shake in the fridge, just for these mornings. You'll want a doughnut, which is why it's so important to have easy access to a shake. If you really, really, really are craving starch and a shake or an omelet just won't do, then have high-fiber cereal. The breakfast that usually fills you up will probably leave you feeling hungry that morning after eating a big dessert. You may even feel hungrier all day long. Eat a larger-than-usual breakfast, if needed, to squelch hunger. If needed, have another shake midmorning.

**Increase your protein portions all day.** If you usually eat 5 ounces, increase them to 8.

**Continue to eat more protein for about a week.** It may take as long as a week for the hunger to subside and the fullness to set back in. It may also take this long for the liver to shed the glycogen and water and for you to see that sudden 5-pound gain reverse itself into a sudden 5-pound drop.

## Lose What You Gain

This is another one of those dirty little secrets about dieting that no one will tell you. Nearly everyone who loses weight gains and reloses many times. They don't lose 60 pounds and keep that 60 pounds off for life. Rather, their weight maintenance resembles the up-and-down rhythm of an EKG readout. They gain 3 pounds, take steps to address it, and then lose 3 pounds. They gain 2 pounds, make another change, and then lose it. They gain 5, and then they lose 5.

They do this over and over again.

If you gain, do the following to turn the numbers around.

**Keep a food log.** One big mistake every day can easily cause weight regain and stoke up your appetite. Many of my patients, during maintenance, ate nearly perfectly all day, but they gained because of one really bad food choice. They reverted to eating bread before dinner instead of after, for example, or they reverted to drinking juice with breakfast. They didn't even realize they had made the change, but they did realize they were hungrier, and didn't know why. They were not eating massive quantities of any one food, but they were eating one fattening food every single day and increasing their overall appetite as a result.

The following foods can be "fattening" because they increase your appetite, making it harder to maintain your weight loss. If you find yourself gaining, write down everything you eat, and look over your records daily and weekly. Look for patterns. What fattening foods have returned to your daily repertoire? Here's a list of common offenders:

- Bread
- Sweets
- Soft drinks
- Juice
- Large servings of pasta
- Large servings of any type of starch, even a whole-grain starch
- Wine or beer before dinner
- Starch before dinner
- Artificial sweeteners
- Fatty foods

**Add more exercise.** Find more ways to sneak in more activity. Can you take a short walk before or after meals? Consider straightening up the house in the evenings instead of reading or watching TV. Ride a bike short distances instead of taking your car.

**Add more vegetables.** Vegetables are the most filling foods on the planet and the best way to reduce your overall calorie intake without feeling as if you are eating less. Look for ways to sneak vegetables into your favorite recipes. Can you add more chopped veggies to your omelet, mushrooms to that burger, or shredded carrots to your meat loaf?

**Get a checkup.** You may be developing diabetes or another health condition, which makes controlling your weight more difficult. You also may have started taking a medicine that is increasing your appetite or slowing your metabolism.

---

You may slip up, regain, and then recommit and lose many times before your weight stays within an even fluctuation. Rather than seeing each small gain as a personal failure, think of small gains as success builders. The more often you get yourself back on track, the stronger you will become. The longer you maintain, the better you will become at maintaining your weight. Research shows that the longer people keep off lost weight, the easier it is for them to maintain. All of their new eating and exercise habits become part of their lives. These habits become so automatic that they rarely think about their food choices. They eat *Skinny* for life.

# Part Four

## Skinny Helpings

# 12

# The Skinny Recipes

n the following pages, you'll find more than fifty recipes that will help you fill up on fewer calories *without* sacrificing flavor. High-satisfaction, low-calorie eating does not have to be synonymous with bland eating. *The Skinny* recipes will show you how to season food with herbs, spices, and other ingredients instead of calorie-laden butter and cream sauces. They'll teach you how to sauté food in chicken or vegetable broth rather than lots of oil. You'll even learn how to create low-calorie sauces and salad dressings that taste just as delicious as their high-calorie counterparts.

I've included dozens of recipes for the types of foods you'll consume day in and day out on the *Skinny* plan. Are you sick of chicken? Sick of fish? Sick of salad? Sick of vegetables? Then consult this chapter—again and again. Here I've provided numerous ways to cook these staples, so you can continually cook *Skinny* meals without hearing your family members complain, "Chicken again?!"

Please note that my recipes are not light on sodium. Salt brings out the flavor of many foods. I'd rather you ate vegetables with a little salt than no vegetables at all. If your physician has recommended that you follow a low-sodium diet, however, please omit the salt in any given recipe—or use a salt substitute.

# Breakfast Dishes

Use the *Skinny* breakfast recipes as a guide to help you create your own *Skinny* omelets and shakes. You are not limited to the three recipes on the following pages. You can combine any assortment of chopped vegetables (bell pepper, spinach, onion, mushroom, and so on) with lean protein (turkey or chicken sausage, roasted turkey breast, lean ham, smoked salmon, crabmeat, and so on) and egg whites to create any number of delicious omelets and frittatas. You can also create your own signature smoothies with nearly any type of frozen fruit (blueberries, melon, peaches, and so on).

## Asparagus Omelet

In this recipe, you'll learn how to use vegetable stock to cut back on high-calorie oils when making omelets.

| | |
|---|---|
| 2 tablespoons plus 1 cup low-sodium vegetable broth | Kosher salt, to taste |
| | Freshly ground black pepper, to taste |
| 4 asparagus spears, sliced into 1-inch pieces | ½ cup baby spinach, stems removed |
| | 3 egg whites |
| ¼ cup sliced cremini ("baby bella") mushrooms | Scant tablespoon finely chopped chives |
| ½ teaspoon minced garlic | 1 teaspoon Dijon mustard |
| ½ teaspoon minced shallot | Nonstick cooking spray |

Put 2 tablespoons broth in an 8- or 10-inch nonstick ovenproof sauté pan over medium-high heat. Add the asparagus and mushrooms and begin stirring. The broth will burn off rather quickly. Continue to cook the vegetables, adding more broth as needed, 2 tablespoons at a time. After 2 to 3 minutes, add the garlic and shallot. Season with salt and pepper. Keep adding broth and stirring the vegetables.

When the asparagus and mushrooms are near done (about 8 minutes), add the spinach and more broth. When the spinach wilts and the broth has cooked off, remove from the heat. Remove the vegetables and wipe the pan.

Whisk the egg whites in a small bowl until frothy. Add the chives and mustard. Whisk to combine.

Spray the sauté pan with nonstick cooking spray and put over medium heat. Add the egg whites, gently swirl the pan once, and reduce the heat to medium-low. Season with salt and pepper to taste. Cook for 4 to 5 minutes.

Preheat the broiler and place the broiler rack about 6 inches from the heat. Place the sauté pan under the broiler for 1 minute. Remove from the broiler and plate the omelet. Lay the reserved vegetables on half the omelet and fold over.

*Serves 1*

## Egg-White Frittata

Frittata keeps well in the refrigerator. Make one a couple of times a week, storing the leftovers in the fridge. Warm them quickly in a toaster oven before eating.

Nonstick cooking spray

One 16-ounce container egg whites or egg substitute

1 tablespoon spice blend (such as lemon pepper or Mediterranean sea salt)

3 scallions, diced and cooked

1 cup shiitake mushrooms, sliced and cooked

4 small turkey sausage links, cooked and sliced

1 ounce shredded reduced-fat cheddar cheese (5 grams of fat or less per ounce)

Preheat the oven to 400°F. Spray an ovenproof skillet with nonstick cooking spray and place it over medium heat. Whisk the egg whites with the spice blend to evenly distribute the spices, then add to the pan. Just as the whites start to set, add the rest of the ingredients, finishing with the cheese. Transfer to the oven and bake for 10 minutes, or until set.

*Serves 4*

## Morning Shake

Most smoothies contain yogurt, ice cream, or some other high-calorie ingredient. This recipe uses water, and, as a result, the entire 2-pint batch will set you back fewer than 300 calories but will keep you feeling full all morning long.

1½ cups frozen strawberries

2 tablespoons ground flaxseed

2 scoops protein powder
(vanilla-flavored seems to work
best)

1 pint water or skim milk

Blend all ingredients until smooth.

*Serves 2*

# Main Dishes

Use main-dish recipes for lunch or for dinner. These recipes will help you learn how to use low-sodium chicken or vegetable broth in place of oil when sautéing food, saving hundreds of extra calories without sacrificing flavor. You'll see that many of these recipes also embed lots of vegetables into the dish to further help you fill up on fewer calories.

## Chef's Salad

2 cups torn romaine leaves

½ medium tomato, cut into wedges

½ green bell pepper, sliced

1 carrot, sliced

½ cup cucumber, sliced

2 ounces cooked skinless turkey
breast, cut into 1-inch strips

1 ounce cooked lean roast beef,
cut into 1-inch strips

2 hard-boiled egg whites, crumbled

Freshly ground black pepper

Mix all of the vegetable ingredients. Sprinkle the turkey, roast beef, and egg whites on top and season with pepper to taste.

*Serves 1*

## Chicken Dijon

4 skinless, boneless chicken breasts,
flattened

¼ cup Dijon mustard

½ cup dry vermouth or white wine

1 tablespoon lemon juice

Freshly ground black pepper

Crushed dried tarragon

Place the chicken breasts in an ovenproof baking dish.

Blend the mustard, vermouth, lemon juice, and pepper to taste in a small mixing bowl. Pour over the chicken and sprinkle with tarragon. Cover and marinate in the refrigerator for at least 1 hour.

Preheat the broiler and place the broiler rack about 6 inches from the heat. Remove the chicken from the marinade and place on the broiler rack. Broil for 5 minutes on each side, basting frequently, until tender.

*Serves 4*

## Chicken Stir-Fry

| | |
|---|---|
| ⅓ cup low-sodium soy sauce | 1 cup thinly sliced carrots |
| 1 tablespoon grated fresh ginger | 1 cup low-sodium chicken broth |
| 1 pound skinless, boneless chicken breasts, cut into 1-inch slices | 1 cup snow peas |
| | 1 cup sliced fresh mushrooms |
| 4 teaspoons olive oil | 1 cup thinly sliced red or green bell peppers |
| 3 garlic cloves, crushed | |
| 2 cups broccoli florets | Salt and pepper |

Mix the soy sauce and ginger in a sealed zip-top bag. Add the chicken and marinate in the refrigerator for several hours.

Heat the olive oil in a large nonstick skillet over medium heat. Add the garlic and sauté for 2 minutes.

Add the chicken with marinade, broccoli, and carrots and cook until the chicken loses its pink color, about 5 to 10 minutes. Add the broth, snow peas, mushrooms, and bell peppers. Cover and reduce the heat to low. Cook for 15 minutes, stirring frequently. Season with salt and pepper to taste.

*Serves 4*

## Chicken Tarragon

| | |
|---|---|
| 1 pound skinless, boneless chicken breasts, trimmed of visible fat | 2 tablespoons fresh or 1 tablespoon dried tarragon |
| ¾ cup low-sodium chicken broth | ⅛ teaspoon freshly ground black pepper |
| ¼ cup lemon juice | |
| 1 teaspoon dry mustard | |

Place the chicken breasts in a baking dish. Mix the broth, lemon juice, mustard, tarragon, and pepper in a small bowl. Pour over the chicken, cover, and marinate in the refrigerator at least 2 hours or overnight.

Preheat the oven to 325°F. Bake for 25 to 30 minutes, or until cooked through.

*Serves 4*

## Fish in Parchment

For this recipe, you'll save on cleanup time by placing a sheet of parchment paper in a baking dish. For ease in serving the fish, lay a smaller piece of parchment in the center of the larger one. You'll be able to lift out this smaller piece, which is more manageable on a plate.

If you're serving this recipe to company, consider zesting the rind of half a lemon over the fish instead of putting lemon slices on it, or squeeze lemon juice on the fish right before serving. Lemon juice kills chlorophyll, so baking the green veggies in lemon juice will turn them a dull color.

| | |
|---|---|
| 12 to 16 asparagus spears, sliced into 1½-inch pieces | 6 tablespoons low-sodium fish broth |
| 16 to 20 haricots verts or green beans, ends trimmed and halved | 2 tablespoons fresh chives, chopped in halves or thirds |
| 1 cup sliced white mushrooms | 2 scant tablespoons roughly chopped fresh tarragon |
| 2 cups torn escarole | 4 thin lemon slices |
| 4 tablespoons thinly sliced shallot or leek | 1 teaspoon chopped fennel fronds, optional |
| Kosher salt | |
| Freshly ground black pepper | |
| 2 fillets whitefish (⅔ pound), such as tilapia, cod, orange roughy, haddock, or flounder | |

Preheat the oven to 400°F and place the rack in the middle of the oven. Place a large piece of parchment paper on top of a shallow casserole dish. Lay the asparagus, haricots verts, mushrooms, escarole, and shallot in a bed in the center of the paper. Sprinkle with salt and pepper to taste.

Lay the fish over the vegetables and season with a pinch of salt and a couple of grinds of pepper. Pour the broth over the fillets. Lay the chives and tarragon on top of the fillets, then top with the lemon slices. Top with fennel fronds, if using.

Gather the short sides of the parchment paper and fold together like the top of a lunch bag. Then fold the sides in, as if wrapping a present.

Bake for 28 to 30 minutes, until the fish flakes easily with a fork. When checking the fish for doneness, be careful when opening the packet, as a lot of steam will build up inside.

Set the packet on a dinner plate and remove the chives, tarragon, lemon slices, and fennel fronds before serving.

*Serves 2*

## Honey Mustard Chicken

| | |
|---|---|
| 1½ tablespoons Dijon or raspberry mustard | 1 pound skinless, boneless chicken breasts, flattened or thinly sliced |
| 1 tablespoon honey | Nonstick cooking spray |
| Freshly ground black pepper | |

Mix the mustard, honey, and pepper in a small bowl. Coat each chicken piece with the mustard mixture. Cover and marinate in the refrigerator for at least 1 hour.

Spray a skillet with nonstick cooking spray and place it over medium heat. Add the chicken and cook, turning occasionally, until it is brown on both sides and cooked through, 5 to 10 minutes.

*Serves 4*

## Marinated Tilapia

Do not marinate fish longer than 30 minutes, or the acid will break down the protein in the fish.

**Marinade:**

| | |
|---|---|
| ½ cup low-sodium fish broth | ⅛ teaspoon kosher salt |
| ¼ cup white wine | ⅛ teaspoon freshly ground black pepper |
| ½ teaspoon lemon zest, grated or cut into strips | |
| 1 teaspoon roughly chopped fresh tarragon | 2 fillets (⅓ pound) tilapia or other medium-fleshed whitefish |
| 1 teaspoon roughly chopped fresh dill | Nonstick cooking spray |

| | |
|---|---|
| 1 teaspoon fresh thyme | ¼ cup panko (Japanese bread |
| 1 tablespoon minced shallot | crumbs), optional |
| 1 teaspoon Dijon mustard | |

Whisk all of the marinade ingredients in a bowl, then pour the marinade into a shallow dish. Bathe both sides of the tilapia in the marinade, then lay the fillets in the dish. Cover and marinate in the refrigerator for 30 minutes.

Preheat the broiler and place the broiler rack about 6 inches below the heat. Line a shallow baking sheet or broiler pan with aluminum foil and spray with nonstick cooking spray. Set the marinated fillets on the baking sheet and spoon some of the marinade on top.

If not using panko, broil the fish 4 minutes on one side, then 3 minutes on the other side. If using panko, then broil the fish 4 to 5 minutes per side. The fish should easily flake with a fork when done. Spread the panko in a dish. Remove the fish from the broiler and coat both sides in the panko. Return to the broiler and broil 1 minute on each side, until golden.

*Serves 2*

## "Noodleless" Spaghetti Pomodoro

| | |
|---|---|
| 1 medium spaghetti squash, cut in | ¼ teaspoon kosher salt |
| half lengthwise and seeded | Freshly ground black pepper, to taste |
| 3 garlic cloves | 1 tablespoon dried oregano |
| 1 teaspoon olive oil | 2 tablespoons grated Parmesan |
| 2 plum or Roma tomatoes, chopped | |
| 2 tablespoons finely chopped fresh | |
| flat-leaf parsley | |

Preheat the oven to 400°F. Fill a baking dish with ¼ to ½ inch water and place the prepared squash halves in it, cut side down. Each half should lie flat in the dish.

Set the garlic on a sheet of aluminum foil and drizzle with the olive oil. Gather the ends of the foil and bring to a close at the top of the garlic, taking care not to rip the foil or leave any openings.

Place the squash and garlic in the oven. Roast the squash until the skin begins to wrinkle, 30 to 35 minutes. Remove the squash and garlic and allow to cool.

When the squash is cool enough to handle, scoop out the flesh from the rind with a fork or spoon, shredding the fibers, and put into a medium bowl. Empty the garlic into a separate small bowl and mash with a fork. Then add the garlic to the squash. Add the tomatoes, parsley, salt, pepper, and oregano to the squash and stir to combine. Sprinkle the Parmesan over the dish and serve.

Variation: Baking imparts a sweeter, more mellow flavor to garlic. If you prefer stronger flavors, sauté the garlic in the oil for 1 to 2 minutes, then add broth to the cooked squash.

*Makes 2 to 3 cups, depending on the size of the squash*

## Poached Salmon

| | |
|---|---|
| 1 pound salmon fillets | 1 bay leaf |
| ¼ cup white wine | 1 celery stalk, quartered |
| 1 small whole onion, quartered | Salt and pepper |
| 2 tablespoons lemon juice | Parsley sprigs |

Bring 2 cups water to a boil in a shallow pan.

Place the salmon in the pan. Add the wine, onion, lemon juice, bay leaf, and celery. Return to a boil, then reduce the heat, cover, and simmer for 10 to 15 minutes. Remove the bay leaf.

Refrigerate and serve cold, seasoned with salt and pepper to taste and garnished with the parsley sprigs.

*Serves 4*

## Pork Chops with Cherry Glaze

If cherries aren't in season, use frozen, no-sugar-added cherries and allow to thaw before cooking.

**Glaze:**

| | |
|---|---|
| 2 cups sweet cherries, pitted | Kosher salt |
| ⅛ cup dry sherry | Freshly ground black pepper |
| 1 tablespoon red wine vinegar or | |
|    balsamic vinegar | 2 boneless pork chops, about 1 inch |
| 4 whole cloves |    thick, trimmed of visible fat |
| Two 2-inch cinnamon sticks | Nonstick cooking spray |

Preheat the oven to 250°F.

Combine the glaze ingredients in a small saucepan and simmer over medium-low heat until reduced by half, about 45 minutes. Remove the cloves and cinnamon sticks.

Liberally salt and pepper both sides of the pork chops. Spray a large nonstick skillet with nonstick cooking spray and place it over medium heat. When it is hot, add the pork chops and sear a few minutes on each side, until brown.

Line a shallow baking dish with aluminum foil and spray with non-stick cooking spray. Bake the seared chops 15 to 20 minutes, until just about cooked through. Pour the reduced glaze and cherries over the chop and bake another 4 to 5 minutes.

*Serves 2*

## Roasted Chicken and Vegetables

A traditional—and easy—method for cooking vegetables with chicken has been to put the vegetables in the cavity of or underneath the bird while it cooks. Because of concerns over salmonella—as well as the addition of fat to the vegetables—this leaner and healthier approach requires roasting the vegetables separately.

¾ cup apple juice or cider

1 tablespoon balsamic vinegar

1 whole chicken (4 to 5 pounds)

1 lemon, halved

Vegetables such as onion, celery, carrot, parsnip, fennel, and garlic, very roughly chopped, optional

Whole fresh herbs, such as thyme, oregano, parsley, and rosemary

Kosher salt

Freshly ground black pepper

3 to 4 cups roasting vegetables, such as sweet potatoes, parsnips, yams, rutabagas, turnips, carrots, fennel, or squash, diced into ½-inch to 1-inch cubes

Preheat the oven to 375°F and place the rack in the middle of the oven.

Whisk the apple juice and balsamic vinegar. Set aside ¼ cup for the chicken and ½ cup for the vegetables. Remove the giblet bag from the chicken cavity. Rinse the inside and outside of the chicken and pat dry, inside and out.

Set the chicken, breast side up, on a rack in a roasting pan and put half of the lemon in the cavity. Add the vegetables, if using, and the fresh herbs. Put the other half of the lemon, rind side out, at the opening of the cavity.

Tuck the wings under the bird and tie the legs together. Season generously with salt and pepper, then brush with ¼ cup marinade.

Roast for 60 minutes, basting every 15 minutes. The chicken skin is going to become very dark and crispy. If it seems on the verge of burning, it's okay to loosely tent foil over the bird, but you must continue to baste it.

Put the roasting vegetables into a bowl and pour ½ cup marinade over them, mixing thoroughly to coat all the vegetables. Pour the vegetables and marinade into a shallow baking pan and spread in one even layer. Season with salt and pepper to taste. Place in the oven next to the chicken.

Roast another 30 minutes, stirring the vegetables occasionally. Check the chicken for doneness. Cut the string on the legs and pull one of the legs—it should release easily and the juices should run clear.

Remove the chicken from the oven and allow it to rest, uncovered, 15 to 20 minutes. Continue to roast the vegetables another 20 to 30 minutes, until tender.

Before carving, tip the chicken to allow the juices to run out of the cavity, transfer the bird to a cutting board or serving dish, and discard the skin and the contents of the cavity.

Variation: Purée the roasted vegetables with chicken or vegetable broth to create a soup.

**Serves 6**


## Salmon Burgers

Note: To toast flaxseeds, place them in a dry skillet over medium heat until fragrant, about 3 to 4 minutes. Then grind them in a coffee grinder for 2 to 3 seconds.

1 cup tightly packed baby spinach leaves, stems removed, rinsed and spun dry

Nonstick cooking spray

Zest of 1 lemon

One 15-ounce can water-packed salmon, deboned and broken into small pieces

| | |
|---|---|
| ½ tablespoon minced garlic | 1 egg |
| ¼ cup finely diced onion | ¼ cup plus 2 tablespoons flaxseeds, |
| ¼ cup low-sodium fish broth | toasted and ground |
| ¼ teaspoon plus ¼ teaspoon kosher | 1 teaspoon chopped fresh dill |
| salt | Olive oil |
| ⅛ teaspoon plus ⅛ teaspoon freshly | |
| ground black pepper | |

Chiffonade the spinach by laying the leaves atop one another and then rolling them up like a cigar, along the long edge. Cut thin strips from one end to the other. Then roughly chop the resulting ribbons.

Spray a frying pan with cooking spray and place it over medium heat. Add the spinach, garlic, onion, broth, ¼ teaspoon salt, and ⅛ teaspoon pepper, and cook until all of the liquid evaporates, about 5 minutes.

Remove the vegetables and transfer them to a medium bowl. Add the lemon zest, salmon, egg, flaxseed, dill, ¼ teaspoon salt, and ⅛ teaspoon pepper. Mix to combine thoroughly. Form burgers to the desired size, creating a slight dimple in the middle on one side.

Brush a grill or grill pan with olive oil, using either a pastry brush or a paper towel, and preheat. Add the burgers, dimple side up, and cook 5 to 7 minutes per side. Try to flip only once. This will help keep them together and retain moistness. Top with salsa, sliced vegetables, or Marinated Grilled Vegetables and Fruit (page 192).

*Makes 3 to 4 burgers*

## Spicy Black Bean Patties

| | |
|---|---|
| 2 teaspoons olive oil | Freshly ground black pepper |
| 3 garlic cloves, minced (about | ¼ cup cornmeal |
| 1 heaping tablespoon) | 1 teaspoon ground cumin |
| ½ white onion, diced | ¼ teaspoon cayenne |
| One 15½-ounce can black beans, | ½ cup cooked brown rice |
| drained and rinsed (reserve some | 1 egg, whisked |
| of the liquid) | Nonstick cooking spray |
| ½ teaspoon kosher salt | |

Heat the olive oil in a nonstick pan over medium-low heat. Add the garlic and onion and cook until softened, stirring frequently, about 8 minutes. Add the beans, salt, and pepper to taste and stir to combine.

Then mash about three fourths of the beans with the back of a wooden spoon, scraping the sides and bottom of the pan. If the beans become dry and begin to stick, add about 1 tablespoon of the bean liquid. The mixture should be pasty, not dry or runny.

When the beans are fully mashed, remove them from the heat and transfer to a medium bowl. Add the cornmeal, cumin, cayenne, and rice to the beans and stir well. When the mixture is cool enough to handle, add the egg and stir or mash with your fingers to combine. Form three or four patties.

Spray a frying pan with nonstick cooking spray and place it over medium heat. Add the patties and cook until golden on one side, about 5 minutes. Give the pan another quick spray when you flip the patties, and cook on the other side until golden.

Serve with red onion, avocado, and tomato on a whole-wheat roll or multigrain English muffin, or top with Pineapple Salsa (page 198).

*Makes 3 palm-sized patties or 4 smaller ones*

## Tangy Flounder or Sole

| | |
|---|---|
| 1¼ pounds flounder or sole fillets (⅛ to ¼ inch thick) | 1 small yellow onion, chopped |
| ¼ cup balsamic vinegar | 2 teaspoons fresh or 1 teaspoon dried parsley |
| ¼ cup lemon juice | Lemon slices, optional |
| 1 teaspoon dry mustard powder | |

Rinse the fish fillets and pat dry. Place the fish in a 10 × 8–inch oven-proof baking dish. Combine the balsamic vinegar, lemon juice, mustard, and onion in a small mixing bowl. Pour over the fillets. Cover and marinate in the refrigerator for up to 30 minutes.

Preheat the broiler. Remove the cover from the dish and broil for 4 to 6 minutes, or until the fish is white and flaky. Garnish with the parsley and lemon slices, if using.

*Serves 4*

## Turkey Chili

| | |
|---|---|
| 1 pound ground white-meat turkey (at least 93% lean) | One 28-ounce can whole tomatoes, undrained and chopped |
| ½ cup chopped onion | 1 to 2 tablespoons chili powder |

| | |
|---|---|
| 2 to 3 cloves garlic, sliced | 1 teaspoon dried oregano |
| One 16-ounce can black beans, rinsed and drained | 1 teaspoon ground cumin |
| | ¼ teaspoon cayenne, optional |
| One 16-ounce can red kidney beans, rinsed and drained | Salt and pepper |

Brown the turkey, onion, and garlic in a nonstick skillet over medium heat, until the meat is no longer pink. Reduce the heat and add the remaining ingredients. Cover and simmer for 15 to 20 minutes.

*Serves 8*

## Zesty Chicken Salad

| | |
|---|---|
| ¼ cup balsamic vinegar | 3 ounces skinless, boneless chicken breast, cooked and cubed |
| 2 tablespoons lemon juice | |
| 1 teaspoon dry mustard | 1 medium tomato, chopped |
| 1 teaspoon dried oregano | 1 large lettuce leaf |

Combine the balsamic vinegar, lemon juice, mustard, and oregano in a small bowl. Place the chicken and tomato in another bowl. Pour the marinade over the chicken and tomato. Cover and marinate in the refrigerator for at least 1 hour.

Serve the cold chicken on top of the lettuce leaf.

*Serves 1*

# Soups and Salads

On this plan, you start lunch and dinner with a soup or salad. What do you do when you've had so many green salads that you can't stand the thought of eating another lettuce leaf? You turn to this section of the book. I've included many different soup and salad recipes to help keep *Skinny* eating interesting.

## Cucumber Salad

This lively salad makes a cooling accompaniment to any spicy main dish. If you use a Kirby cucumber in this salad, seed it by running a spoon down the center.

| | |
|---|---|
| 1 medium cucumber, peeled and thinly sliced | A few shaves of lime zest |
| ⅔ cup thinly sliced red onion | 4 tablespoons plain low-fat or nonfat yogurt |
| 2 tablespoons roughly chopped fresh cilantro | Dash of kosher salt |
| | A few grinds of black pepper |

Mix all of the ingredients in a small bowl. Serve immediately.
*Serves 2*

## Easiest Vegetable Soup

| | |
|---|---|
| 4 cups low-sodium vegetable broth | 2 garlic cloves, minced |
| 4 carrots, cut diagonally into coins | 1 bay leaf |
| 4 celery stalks, cut into ½-inch slices (leaves okay) | 1 teaspoon kosher salt |
| ½ small onion, diced | Freshly ground black pepper |
| | Chopped fresh flat-leaf parsley |

Heat ½ cup broth in a soup pot over medium-high heat. Add the carrots, celery, and onion. Cook, stirring periodically, then add another ½ cup stock when the pot is almost dry. Add the garlic, bay leaf, salt, and pepper to taste.

Continue to cook, stirring periodically. Add the final 3 cups stock when the pot is almost dry. (The carrots should just be starting to soften.) Reduce the heat to low, cover, and simmer for about 30 minutes, until the vegetables are tender.

Remove the bay leaf and serve the soup with a sprinkling of parsley.

Variation: You can easily modify this into a chicken soup recipe by substituting chicken broth for the vegetable broth. Bring all 4 cups of broth to a boil. Add 1 or 2 boneless, skinless chicken breasts, cover, reduce the heat, and simmer 5 to 6 minutes. Remove the pot from the heat, cover, and set aside. Cook chicken in the hot broth until done, about 15 minutes. When done, remove the chicken from the stock and set aside to cool. Skim the fat from the top of the stock, then follow the Easiest Vegetable Soup recipe, using the remaining stock. When the chicken is cool, shred it and add it to the soup at the end, about 5 minutes before the vegetables are done, to heat the chicken through.

You may also add other soup vegetables, such as mushrooms, bok choy, and cabbage, as well as your favorite spices.

*Makes 1 quart*

## Gazpacho

3½ cups chopped tomatoes (about 4), or one 28-ounce can diced tomatoes

1 cup chopped cucumber (about 1 medium), peeled, cut lengthwise, and seeded, or seedless

⅓ cup diced red onion

1 cup diced yellow bell pepper (about 1 small)

½ serrano pepper, seeded and minced (if less heat is desired, use a jalapeño instead)

1 tablespoon red wine vinegar

Juice of 2 small limes

½ cup low-sodium tomato juice or vegetable juice blend

8 grinds of black pepper

1 teaspoon kosher salt

Minced garlic, optional

1 tablespoon roughly chopped fresh cilantro

Plain low-fat or nonfat yogurt

Mix all of the ingredients except the cilantro and yogurt in a medium bowl. (For a less rustic version, blend half of the soup in a blender, or use an immersion blender to purée about half of the soup while in the bowl.) Stir in the cilantro. Cover and refrigerate until chilled. Before serving, top each bowl with a dollop of yogurt.

*Makes 4 cups*

## Lentil Soup

This recipe calls for brown lentils. If you prefer red lentils, halve the cooking time. Brown lentils hold their shape better, making them a good option if you prefer chunkier, unpuréed soup. Note: If you have only iodized salt, omit the salt altogether. It will lend an overly salty flavor to the recipe.

½ cup plus 3 cups low-sodium vegetable or chicken broth

½ cup finely diced carrot

⅓ cup finely diced celery

½ teaspoon cumin

½ teaspoon coriander

Pinch of kosher salt

Freshly ground black pepper

½ cup finely diced onion

1½ to 2 teaspoons minced garlic

1 tablespoon red wine vinegar

1 bay leaf

1 large thyme sprig

½ teaspoon celery salt

½ to ¾ cup brown lentils, picked over
   and rinsed

½ tomato, seeded and chopped
   (about ½ cup)

Plain nonfat yogurt or Simple Pepper
   Coulis (page 199), optional

Heat ½ cup broth in a soup pot over medium-high heat. Add the carrot, celery, and onion. Cook, stirring occasionally, for 5 minutes. Add the garlic. Cook for 4 to 5 minutes more, and just before the broth evaporates, reduce the heat to medium-low. Stir often, keeping an eye on it so the vegetables don't brown or stick to the bottom. When the liquid is gone, cook another 1 to 2 minutes, stirring constantly to keep the vegetables from sticking.

Add the vinegar and stir another minute or so. Add 3 cups broth and the bay leaf, thyme, celery salt, cumin, coriander, salt, and pepper to taste.

When the broth is hot, add the lentils and tomato. Cook until the lentils are soft and split open, 30 to 35 minutes. If too much liquid evaporates, reduce the heat after 20 minutes and partially cover the pot. You may also add more broth, ½ cup at a time, if desired.

Remove the bay leaf and thyme sprig before serving. Serve as is, or purée in a blender or with an immersion blender. If puréed, serve the soup with a swirl of yogurt or coulis.

*Makes 1 quart*

## Orange, Radish, and Roasted Asparagus Salad

Select asparagus spears with closed tips, as open ones may scorch under the broiler.

**Dressing:**

1 tablespoon Orange Oil (page 197)

½ tablespoon apple cider vinegar

¼ teaspoon Dijon mustard

Kosher salt

Freshly ground black pepper

8 thin asparagus spears

1 tablespoon pine nuts

1½ cups packed baby spinach leaves,
   stems removed, rinsed and spun
   dry

1 radish, thinly sliced

A few curls of Parmesan, shaved off
   a block with a vegetable peeler

Nonstick cooking spray
½ minneola, tangelo, or other small,
    juicy orange citrus fruit

Whisk all the dressing ingredients. Set aside.

Preheat the broiler and place the broiler rack about 4 inches below the heat. Line a shallow broiling pan with aluminum foil and spray gently with nonstick cooking spray. Roll the asparagus around the pan to coat with spray, then put it under the broiler. Broil, turning once, about 4 minutes, until done. (The asparagus may also be grilled.) Once the spears are cooked, cut them into 1-inch pieces, discarding the bottom inch.

Cut the orange in half crosswise, then remove the skin and the pith with a sharp knife. Separate the peeled sections and cut them into chunks.

Toast the pine nuts in a dry pan over medium heat until just golden and fragrant, shaking the pan occasionally, 6 to 8 minutes.

Toss the spinach with the asparagus, orange, and radish. Add dressing. Top with the pine nuts and Parmesan.

You can turn this starter salad into a full meal by adding chicken. Pound 1 boneless, skinless chicken breast flat. Season with salt and pepper to taste, then brush with the reserved half of the dressing. Marinate in the refrigerator for 15 to 30 minutes. Meanwhile, preheat the oven to 350°F. Line a shallow baking pan with aluminum foil, spray with nonstick cooking spray, add the chicken, and bake 20 to 30 minutes, depending on the size and thickness of the breast, until done. Either serve the chicken alongside the salad, or slice it when cool enough to handle and add it to the salad.

*Serves 1*

## Pomegranate Salad

You can turn this starter salad into a full meal by omitting the toppings and using the dressed greens as a bed for seared scallops, broiled skirt steak, or grilled pork loin.

**Dressing:**

1 tablespoon Pomegranate Oil          4 cups packed baby arugula, washed
    (page 197)                             and spun dry

2 tablespoons red wine vinegar

1 tablespoon honey

kosher salt

Freshly ground black pepper

2 teaspoons lemon juice

1 tablespoon chopped shallots, plus
  more sliced, if desired

¼ cup chopped walnuts

A few curls of Parmesan, shaved off a
  block with a vegetable peeler

A handful of pomegranate seeds, if in
  season, optional

Whisk the dressing ingredients. Set aside.

Place the arugula in a bowl and toss with dressing. Top with the walnuts and Parmesan and the pomegranate seeds and sliced shallots, if using.

*Serves 3 to 4*

## Strawberry-Spinach Salad

**Dressing:**

1 tablespoon Balsamic Strawberry
  Sauce (page 195)

¼ to ½ teaspoon poppy seeds

1 tablespoon chopped hazelnuts

1½ cups packed baby spinach leaves,
  stems removed, rinsed and spun
  dry

1 tablespoon sliced red onion or
  shallot

¼ cup hothouse cucumber (or Kirby
  cucumber, seeded), cut in half and
  thinly sliced (about ½ medium)

A few curls of Parmesan, shaved off a
  block with a vegetable peeler

A handful of small strawberries,
  optional

Combine the dressing ingredients. Set aside.

Toast the hazelnuts in a dry pan over medium heat until just golden and fragrant, shaking the pan occasionally, 6 to 8 minutes.

Toss the spinach with the onion and cucumber. Add the dressing. Top with the hazelnuts and Parmesan. Garnish with the strawberries, if using.

*Serves 1*

## Tuna Salad

4 ounces water-packed tuna, drained

1 tablespoon reduced-fat mayonnaise

1 teaspoon red wine vinegar

Freshly ground black pepper

| 1 celery stalk, chopped | Garlic powder |
| 1 scallion, chopped | |

Mix all of the ingredients in a small bowl. Serve over salad greens.
*Serves 1*

## Tuscan White Bean Soup

This recipe makes more than a quart of soup, but it freezes well. Allow it to cool, pour into containers to cool it completely in the fridge, then freeze. For an even heartier soup, add chopped cubes of thick-cut lean ham.

| | |
|---|---|
| 5 cups low-sodium vegetable or chicken broth | 2 tablespoons chopped garlic (2 to 4 cloves) |
| 3 to 4 carrots, cut diagonally into coins (about 2 cups) | ½ cup white wine, such as Pinot Grigio |
| 4 celery stalks, thinly sliced (about 2 cups) | Two 15½-ounce cans cannellini or great northern beans, drained and rinsed |
| 1 medium white onion, diced (about 2 cups) | 4 cups packed escarole (about 1 small head), large leaves cut in half |
| 4 or 5 fresh thyme sprigs | Grated Parmesan, optional |
| 2 fresh oregano sprigs | Chopped fresh flat-leaf parsley, optional |
| 1 bay leaf | |
| ½ tablespoon kosher salt, plus more to taste | |
| ½ teaspoon freshly ground black pepper, plus more to taste | |

Pour 1 cup broth into a large soup pot over medium-high heat. When the broth is hot, add the carrots, celery, and onion. Stir to combine, then reduce the heat to medium. Cook for 5 minutes, then add the thyme, oregano, bay leaf, salt, and pepper. Cook for another 5 minutes, then add the garlic. Continue to sweat the vegetables until the liquid is nearly evaporated, stirring occasionally, about 25 minutes.

Increase the heat to high, then add the wine. Stir frequently, scraping the bottom of the pot, until the liquid is evaporated, 2 to 3 minutes. When it seems as if the vegetables are going to stick to the bottom of the pan because there's no liquid left, add the rest of the broth and reduce the heat to medium-low.

Remove the thyme, oregano, and bay leaf. Add the beans and escarole. Add salt and pepper to taste.

Simmer for 30 minutes. Serve with Parmesan and parsley, if using.
*Makes a bit more than 1 quart*

## Vegetable Salad

| | |
|---|---|
| 1 cup torn romaine leaves | 1 large carrot, sliced |
| 1 cup torn green or red leaf lettuce leaves | 5 fresh mushrooms, sliced |
| | ½ cucumber, sliced |
| 1 medium tomato, sliced | 1 tablespoon chopped onion |
| ½ red bell pepper, sliced | Freshly ground black pepper |

Place all of the ingredients in a large wooden salad bowl and toss.
*Serves 1*

# Vegetable Side Dishes

If you don't want to spend a lot of time in the kitchen, I encourage you to use any number of steam-in-a-bag products now available at most grocery stores. I've provided a list of great brands on page 203. If you enjoy cooking, however, I've included many recipes in the following pages to accompany your main course.

## Balsamic Portabella Mushrooms

| | |
|---|---|
| 2 portabella mushroom caps | ¼ teaspoon kosher salt |
| ¼ cup balsamic vinegar | Freshly ground black pepper |
| 1 tablespoon olive oil | Chopped fresh flat-leaf parsley |
| 1 tablespoon minced garlic | |

Clean the mushroom caps with a paper towel. Lay them in a shallow baking dish, gills down.

Whisk the balsamic vinegar, olive oil, garlic, salt, and pepper to taste in a small bowl. Pour the marinade over the mushrooms, spooning the mixture to ensure that the entire cap gets coated. Flip the caps over and spoon the marinade into the gills; allow some marinade to remain in the bottom of the dish to keep the tops of the caps moist. Set aside for 10 to 15 minutes.

Preheat the broiler and place the broiler rack about 6 inches below the heat. Flip the caps over, gills down, and broil for 2 minutes. Flip over and broil for another 2 minutes. Remove to a plate and sprinkle with parsley.

*Makes 2 caps*

## Curried Cauliflower

| | |
|---|---|
| 2 teaspoons olive oil | ¼ teaspoon ground cinnamon |
| 1 head cauliflower, cut into bite-sized | ⅛ teaspoon ground allspice |
| florets | ¼ teaspoon kosher salt |
| ½ cup chopped white onion | Freshly ground black pepper |
| 1½ cups low-sodium vegetable broth | 1 tablespoon minced garlic (about |
| ½ teaspoon curry powder | 1 clove) |
| ¼ teaspoon ground cumin | 1 teaspoon minced jalapeño |

Heat the olive oil in a large skillet over medium heat. Add the cauliflower and the onion and stir to coat with the oil. Cook, stirring occasionally, until the onion starts to brown and turn translucent, 5 to 10 minutes. Add the broth and increase the heat to medium-high. Add the curry powder, cumin, cinnamon, allspice, salt, and pepper to taste. Stir to combine, then simmer about 8 minutes, stirring occasionally. If the liquid begins to boil, reduce the heat to medium. Add the garlic and the jalapeño, stir to combine, then cook, stirring occasionally, until the cauliflower softens and almost all of the liquid evaporates, 5 to 10 minutes. Give it a final stir and serve.

*Makes 3 to 4 cups, depending on the size of the florets*

## Green Beans with Escarole

Do not put the escarole into a salad spinner or dry it off; retain as much of the water as possible on the leaves after rinsing.

| | |
|---|---|
| Kosher salt | 1 teaspoon lemon zest |
| ¾ pound fresh green beans, picked | Freshly ground black pepper |
| over, ends trimmed | Chopped fresh flat-leaf parsley, |
| 1 teaspoon olive oil | optional |

1 large garlic clove, minced

1-pound head escarole, rinsed and
  cored

Bring a medium pot of water, ¾ full, with ½ teaspoon salt, to a boil.

Add the green beans to the boiling water and cook until bright green, 5 to 8 minutes. Drain and set aside.

Heat the olive oil in a large skillet over medium heat. Add the garlic and cook, stirring, until fragrant, about 1 minute. Remove the garlic and set it aside. Wipe the pan with a paper towel.

Return the pan to medium heat. Add the escarole and salt to taste, stirring to distribute the moisture and salt. Reduce the heat to medium-low and cook, stirring occasionally, until the leaves are wilted, 5 to 6 minutes. When the escarole is wilted, add the garlic, green beans, lemon zest, and pepper to taste. Stir to combine and heat through. Sprinkle with parsley, if using, and serve.

*Serves 2; makes 3 cups*

## Jicama Slaw

Serve as a refreshing and light alternative to traditional coleslaw, or eat as a satisfying between-meals snack.

1 pound jicama

3 medium carrots

¼ teaspoon kosher salt

¼ teaspoon freshly ground black
  pepper

1 Granny Smith apple

Juice of ½ lime

Peel the jicama with a paring knife or vegetable peeler. Cut into matchsticks, halving the longer sticks. Put the sticks into a medium bowl. Peel the carrots and cut into matchsticks. Add to the bowl. Add the salt and pepper and mix the jicama and carrot sticks to distribute the seasonings. Cut two opposite sides off the apple, cutting close to the core. Lay each side cut-side down and slice thinly, keeping the peel on. Add to the bowl. Add the lime juice and mix to combine.

*Serves 2; makes about 5 cups*

## Marinated Grilled Vegetables and Fruit

Good grilling vegetables include yellow and green summer squash, eggplant, baby bok choy, and portabella mushrooms. If you are using vegetables with leaves (such as bok choy), trim any excess leaves if using an open flame.

**Dipping sauce:**

½ cup nonfat yogurt

2 teaspoons honey

½ teaspoon lime juice

**Marinade:**

1 tablespoon low-sodium soy sauce

1 tablespoon brown rice vinegar

1 tablespoon olive oil

Salt and pepper

2 cups sliced fruit (such as peaches, plums, and pineapple)

2 cups vegetables, cut into uniform pieces

Mix the dipping sauce ingredients in a small bowl. Set aside.

Preheat a grill or grill pan. Mix the marinade ingredients in a small bowl. Place the vegetables in the marinade, and then set them on the grill. Sprinkle with salt and pepper to taste and grill until there are grill marks on each side.

Grill the sliced fruit until there are grill marks on each side. Serve with dipping sauce.

*Serves 1 to 2*

## Mushroom Sauté

Kosher salt does not have iodine added to it, so it has a cleaner—and saltier—taste. The flakes are larger than iodized salt granules, so a portion of kosher salt has half the sodium of an equal portion of iodized salt. If using iodized salt in this recipe, use half the amount.

½ cup plus ½ cup low-sodium vegetable broth

16 ounces sliced cremini ("baby bella") mushrooms

2 tablespoons balsamic vinegar

2½ to 4 tablespoons roughly chopped fresh flat-leaf parsley

Juice of 1 small lemon

| 6 scallions, white and light green | ½ teaspoon kosher salt |
| parts (about ¼ cup) | Freshly ground black pepper |
| 4 garlic cloves, minced | 2 tablespoons white wine |

Put ½ cup broth in a small frying pan over medium-high heat and cook until it begins to sizzle, then add the mushrooms. Stir occasionally.

When the liquid has almost totally evaporated, add the scallions and garlic and ½ cup broth. Stir occasionally, scraping the bottom of the pan. When the liquid has evaporated again, reduce the heat to low and add the balsamic vinegar, parsley, lemon juice, salt, and pepper to taste. Stir to blend and burn off the vinegar.

Increase the heat to high, add the wine, and cook, stirring constantly, scraping the bottom of the pan, until the liquid has evaporated.

*Serves 2*

## Roasted Vegetables

| Roasting vegetables (Brussels | 1 teaspoon olive oil |
| sprouts, asparagus, broccoli | Your favorite spice blend |
| florets, artichokes, onions, | Nonstick cooking spray |
| eggplant, and fennel) | |

Preheat the oven to 400° F. Cut the vegetables into even pieces. This allows them to cook evenly. Place them in a zip-top bag with the olive oil and spice blend to taste. Shake to thoroughly coat the vegetables.

Spray a casserole dish with nonstick cooking spray and add the vegetables. Roast until tender and slightly browned (cooking time will vary by vegetable), stirring a few times.

*Serves 1 or more*

## Spicy Kale with Garlic Chips

| 2 large garlic cloves | ¼ teaspoon kosher salt |
| ½ tablespoon olive oil | 1 teaspoon lemon juice |
| 1 medium bunch kale, roughly | ¼ teaspoon crushed red pepper |
| chopped | flakes |

Thinly slice the garlic crosswise, to create "chips" about ⅛ inch thick.

Heat the olive oil in a large skillet over medium heat. Add the garlic. Don't stir. Cook until it begins to sizzle and just starts to brown, 2 to 3 minutes. Remove the garlic and set it aside. Wipe the pan with a paper towel.

Rinse the kale, leaving much of the moisture on it. Add the kale and the salt to the pan, stirring to coat the kale. When the kale begins to uniformly wilt, 3 to 5 minutes, reduce the heat to medium-low.

Add the lemon juice to the kale and stir to coat. Cook for 1 minute. Return the garlic to the pan and add the red pepper flakes. Stir to combine, and serve.

*Makes 2 cups*

## Sauces and Dressings

Salad dressings and sauces can add hundreds of extra calories from fat and sugar to a dish. In comparison, the recipes in the following pages are light in calories, but they are heavy in satisfaction. They are just as flavorful as their higher-calorie cousins. In addition to these sauces and dressings, consider flavoring food with the following low- or no-calorie ingredients:

**Spice rubs and spice blends:** Use them on fish and meat or even sprinkle them over salads and other dishes for extra flavor. Experiment with various blends such as lemon pepper or Mediterranean sea salt, or try the following spice combinations:

- Coriander, paprika, chili powder
- Brown sugar, kosher salt, cumin, black pepper, garlic powder, paprika, chili powder, ancho chili powder
- Cumin, paprika, chili powder, coriander, curry powder, cayenne, black pepper, kosher salt

**Salsa:** Use the Salsa Verde recipe (page 198) or commercially prepared salsa to top fish, burgers, and even salads. At roughly 15 calories per 2 tablespoons, you can't overdo it.

**Flavored vinegar:** Try rice wine vinegar, garlic vinegar, or another flavor over salads, along with your favorite spice blend. Vinegar adds very few calories to your dish but lots of flavor, and it also helps slow digestion and improve your sense of fullness.

**Mustard:** You'll find mustard used in many of the dressings in the following pages for a reason. An entire tablespoon contains only about 15 calories, depending on the type of mustard. Compare that to mayonnaise's 110 calories per tablespoon and you can see how this one switch can save you lots of calories without sacrificing flavor.

## Apple Cider Dressing

¼ cup apple cider vinegar

3 tablespoons lemon juice

2 teaspoons artificial sweetener

1 teaspoon dry mustard

1 teaspoon celery seed

Whisk all of the ingredients in a small bowl.

*Makes ½ cup; 1½ tablespoons per serving*

## Balsamic Strawberry Sauce

The finished sauce makes a lovely accompaniment to lamb—simply dollop it on the meat prior to serving; it can also be used for salad dressing.

1 cup fresh or frozen strawberries, hulled and quartered

½ teaspoon sugar or Splenda

1 tablespoon balsamic vinegar

2 grinds of black pepper

Combine all of the ingredients in a small bowl, and stir gently. Set aside for 30 minutes.

Heat a saucepan over low heat. Add the strawberry mixture and cook for 10 minutes. When it starts to bubble, begin stirring gently and continuously. Remove from the heat and cool slightly while still stirring.

Place the mixture in a blender or food processor, or use an immersion blender, and purée on low speed until smooth. Cover and refrigerate until ready to use.

*Makes about ½ cup; 1½ tablespoons per serving*

## Dijon Dressing

2 tablespoons canola oil

6 tablespoons red wine vinegar

2 cloves garlic, minced

2 tablespoons Dijon mustard

Whisk all of the ingredients in a small bowl.

*Makes ¾ cup; 1½ tablespoons per serving*

## Guacamole

Guacamole goes well with tacos, particularly fish tacos. Also use it to top chicken or fish. Seed the tomato by slicing it, scraping out the seeds and liquid, *then* chopping.

1 ripe Hass avocado, peeled and
  roughly chopped
2 tablespoons fresh lime juice
1 teaspoon chopped garlic

¼ teaspoon kosher salt
1 tablespoon chopped fresh cilantro
⅓ cup seeded, chopped tomato

Mash the avocado with the lime juice until the avocado is the desired consistency (creamy or chunky). On a cutting board, mash the garlic with the salt to form a paste, then add to the avocado-lime mixture along with the cilantro. Add the tomato to the other ingredients and mix until combined.

*Makes 1 cup; 1 tablespoon per serving*

## Lemon Yogurt Dressing

½ cup plain nonfat yogurt
Juice of 1 lemon and finely chopped
  zest
½ clove garlic, minced

¼ teaspoon chopped fresh parsley or
  ⅛ teaspoon dried parsley
Freshly ground black pepper

Whisk all of the ingredients in a small bowl.

*Makes ½ cup; 1 tablespoon per serving*

## Low-Calorie Vinaigrette

2 tablespoons olive oil
3 tablespoons balsamic vinegar
3 tablespoons rice vinegar

¼ teaspoon kosher salt
Freshly ground black pepper
Minced garlic

Whisk all of the ingredients in a small bowl.

*Makes ½ cup; 1½ tablespoons per serving*

## Orange Oil

This oil can be used as a fat-free base for salad dressings, sauces, and marinades.

1 cup pure orange juice (no sugar
   added, not from concentrate)

Strain the orange juice through a fine mesh sieve or damp cheese-cloth to remove all pulp. Place in a small saucepan over medium-low heat, until just about to boil. Reduce the heat to low and simmer, stirring occasionally and skimming any solids that form on the top of the juice. Cook the juice down and reduce it until thick and smooth. When the juice begins to bubble and percolate, lower the heat and stir more frequently. Cook until you can tilt the saucepan and the oil is thick enough to coat the bottom, about 90 minutes. Pour into a separate container and set aside until it stops steaming and the container is cool to the touch. Cover and refrigerate until ready to use.

*Serving size = 1 tablespoon*

## Pico de Gallo

Though pico de gallo is essentially just another name for salsa, it can be used to top grilled chicken or fish or Spicy Black Bean Patties (page 180).

3 Roma or plum tomatoes, seeded
   and chopped
½ small red onion, finely chopped
   (about ½ cup)
2 tablespoons chopped fresh cilantro

½ teaspoon kosher salt
1½ tablespoons lime juice
½ serrano pepper, seeded and
   minced

Mix all of the ingredients in a bowl.

*Makes 1 cup; 1 or more servings*

## Pomegranate Oil

Use this oil as a fat-free base for salad dressings, sauces, and marinades.

1 cup pure pomegranate juice (no
   sugar added and preferably not
   from concentrate)

If squeezing fresh pomegranate juice, strain the juice through a fine mesh sieve or a damp cheesecloth to remove all the pith. Place the juice in a small saucepan over medium-low heat and simmer for about an hour, stirring occasionally. Cook until you can tilt the saucepan and the oil is thick enough to still coat the bottom. Pour into a separate container and set aside until it stops steaming and the container is cool to the touch. Cover and refrigerate until ready to use.

*Serving size = 1 tablespoon*

## Pineapple Salsa

This salsa is a perfect topper for Spicy Black Bean Patties (page 180), grilled chicken, steamed whitefish, or broiled shrimp.

2 cups diced pineapple, drained (or about ¼ whole pineapple, peeled, cored, and chopped)

1 teaspoon minced jalapeño (about ¼ pepper—add up to ½ pepper if more heat is desired), seeded

¾ cup diced red bell pepper (about ½ medium pepper)

¼ cup finely chopped red onion (about ½ small onion)

4 teaspoons freshly squeezed lime juice (about 1 lime, depending on size)

Pinch of kosher salt

2 tablespoons roughly chopped fresh cilantro (stems are supple enough to be included)

Place all of the ingredients in a medium bowl and stir to combine. Cover and set aside; for immediate use or refrigerate to blend the flavors.

*Makes about 3 cups; 3 or more servings*

## Salsa Verde

Salsa verde is excellent over scrambled eggs, omelets, or taco meat.

Nonstick cooking spray

2 cups whole tomatillos, husked and washed of their sticky residue

1 cup low-sodium vegetable broth

½ cup chopped onion

1 tablespoon chopped garlic

1 jalapeño, seeded and chopped (or use a serrano for more heat)

Kosher salt

½ tablespoon chopped fresh cilantro

Preheat the oven to 400° F. Line a shallow baking pan with aluminum foil and spray with nonstick cooking spray. Set the tomatillos in the pan and bake about 15 minutes, until golden and wrinkly. Remove from the oven, and when they are cool enough to handle, roughly chop them.

Heat the broth in a medium saucepan over medium-high heat, then add the onion, garlic, jalapeño, and ¼ teaspoon salt. Stir occasionally. Just before the broth completely evaporates, remove the pan from the heat and add the tomatillos, cilantro, and more salt to taste. Mix to combine. If the salsa is too soupy, return it to the heat to evaporate some of the liquid.

*Makes 1½ cups; 1 or more servings*

## Simple Pepper Coulis

Coulis are simply puréed fruits or vegetables, and you can make low-calorie coulis with just about any vegetable. Sweat the vegetable in a bit of vegetable broth and your favorite herbs (garlic, salt and pepper, basil, and so on) until very tender, then purée. Or roast a vegetable, as in this recipe. Serve over burgers, chicken breasts, steaks or chops, fish, pasta, or grilled portabella mushrooms. It can even be used in place of mayonnaise as a spread. For example, purée a roasted yellow pepper with a bit of fresh ginger, and you have a great topper for grilled tuna. Roast tomatoes and garlic and purée with a bit of basil for a thin tomato sauce.

1 medium to large red, orange, or
   yellow bell pepper

Trim any excess stem, but keep the pepper intact. Turn a gas burner to medium-high heat or set the rack of a grill directly among the coals. Lay the pepper directly on the burner grate or grill rack and roast it in the flame. As the skin begins to scorch, turn the pepper over with tongs. Keep turning it periodically, and move the pepper around for even roasting, though there's no need to thoroughly blacken the entire pepper. When done, place the pepper in a zip-top bag, seal it, and allow to stand, about 10 minutes.

Remove the pepper from the bag. When it's cool enough to handle, remove the skin. Seed the pepper by cutting around the stem first. Then chop it into large chunks. Put it into a blender or small food processor and purée until smooth.

*Makes ⅓ to ½ cups; 1½ tablespoons per serving*

## Tomato, Artichoke, and Caper Relish

This relish goes great with fish (such as salmon, tilapia, or turbot) and chicken. It makes enough to cover one fillet or cutlet.

10 basil leaves

1 pint grape or cherry tomatoes, cut in half

½ cup canned artichoke hearts in water (about 8 quarters)

2 tablespoons nonpareille capers, drained but not rinsed

Pinch of kosher salt

Freshly ground black pepper

1 teaspoon lemon juice

1 tablespoon grated Parmesan

Chiffonade the basil by laying the leaves atop one another and then rolling them up like a cigar, along the long edge. Cut thin strips from one end to the other.

Mix the basil with the rest of the ingredients in a bowl. Serve meat or fish with the relish on top.

*Makes 2 cups*

## Yogurt Dill Sauce

Serve this easy sauce over fish, especially salmon.

1 teaspoon Dijon mustard

1 cup plain nonfat yogurt

2 tablespoons chopped fresh dill

Mix the mustard and yogurt. Add the dill and thoroughly combine.

*Makes 1 cup; 1 tablespoon per serving*

# Skinny Resources

n this section, I've included everything you need to follow *The Skinny* for life.

## Skinny Recommended Frozen Dinners

Look for dinners with 250 to 350 calories, fewer than 10 grams of fat, fewer than 30 grams of carbohydrate, 3 grams of fiber or more, fewer than 8 grams of sugar, and more than 15 grams of protein. The following brands meet those criteria:

**Lean Cuisine**
  Baked Chicken Florentine
  Chicken in Peanut Sauce
  Fiesta Grilled Chicken
  Garlic Beef and Broccoli
  Lemongrass Chicken
  Meatloaf with Gravy and Whipped Potatoes

Salisbury Steak with Macaroni and Cheese
Steak Tips Portabello

**Smart Ones**
Meatloaf
Salisbury Steak

**Kashi**
Chicken Florentine

**South Beach Living**
Roasted Turkey
Caprese Style Chicken
Garlic Herb Chicken
Meatloaf with Gravy
Garlic Parmesan Chicken
Savory Beef
Savory Pork

**Gorton's**
Garlic Butter Grilled Fillets
Cajun Blackened Grilled Fillets
Classic Chargrilled Fillets

## Skinny Recommended Grains

The following whole-grain brands offer at least 2 grams of fiber per serving. Whenever possible, choose the highest-fiber grain available.

Arnold
Aunt Millie's
Baker's Inn
Healthy Life
Nature's Own
Rudi's Organic Bakery
Thomas' Light English Muffins
Mission Foods wraps

## Skinny Recommended Vegetable Brands

Steam-in-a-bag and frozen vegetables provide convenient ways to get in your vegetable servings. Look for any variety that does not come with a sauce. Recommended brands include the following:

Green Giant Simply Steam and Frozen Select frozen vegetables
Birds Eye frozen vegetables and Steamfresh vegetables
Cascadian Farms frozen vegetables

## Skinny Recommended Fruit and Vegetable Varieties

The fruits and vegetables in the following lists are all low in GL (see p. 208), so they are least likely to trigger rebound hunger. Choose fresh or frozen without sugar added. Berries, melons, and apples affect your blood sugar the least.

**Fruits**
Apples
Apricots
Blackberries
Blueberries
Cantaloupe
Cherries
Grapefruit
Honeydew
Kiwifruit
Mangoes
Oranges
Peaches
Pears
Pineapples
Plums
Raspberries
Strawberries
Tangerines
Watermelon

**Vegetables**
  Artichokes
  Asparagus
  Beets
  Broccoli
  Cabbage
  Cauliflower

## Skinny Recommended Frozen Desserts

The following desserts all come in individual portions and take a long time to eat, helping to prevent overeating. (Note: A product containing sugar alcohols may give gastric distress.)

| Product | Calories | Fat (g) |
|---|---|---|
| Popsicle—Sugar Free Popsicles (1 pop) | 15 | 0 |
| Breyers—All Natural Ice Cream | 140 | 8 |
| Tofutti—Chocolate Fudge Treats | 30 | 0 |
| Edy's—Fruit Bars No Sugar Added | 30 | 0 |
| Popsicle—No Sugar Added Fudgsicle (2 pops) | 80 | 1.5 |
| Edy's—Orange and Cream Fruit Bars | 80 | 1.5 |
| Häagen-Dazs—Fat Free Sorbet & Yogurt Bars | 90 | 0 |
| Nestlé—Minis Ice Cream Sandwiches | 90 | 3 |
| Skinny Cow—Low-Fat Fudge Bar | 100 | 1 |
| Edy's—Real Fruit Smoothie & Yogurt | 100 | 2 |
| Skinny Cow—Mini Fudge Bars | 100 | 2 |
| Skinny Cow—Low Fat Ice Cream Bar | 120 | 0.5 |
| Tofutti—Cuties | 120 | 5 |
| Weight Watchers—Chocolate Mousse Ice Cream Bar (2 bars) | 120 | 1 |

Celery
Cucumbers
Eggplant
Green beans
Mushrooms
Onions
Peppers
Scallions
Spaghetti squash
Spinach
Tomatoes
Yellow squash
Zucchini

| Saturated Fat (g) | Carbs (g) | Fiber (g) | Sugars (g) | Sugar Alcohols (g) |
|---|---|---|---|---|
| 0 | 4 | 0 | 0 | 2 |
| 4.5 | 16 | 0 | 14 | 0 |
| 0 | 6 | 0 | 0 | 4 |
| 0 | 8 | 0 | 2 | 2 |
| 1.5 | 18 | 4 | 5 | 4 |
| 0.5 | 16 | 0 | 15 | 0 |
| 0 | 21 | 0 | 15 | 0 |
| 2 | 14 | 0 | 7 | 0 |
| 0.5 | 22 | 4 | 13 | 0 |
| 1 | 18 | 3 | 13 | 0 |
| 1 | 19 | 1 | 7 | 5 |
| 0.5 | 23 | 2 | 15 | 0 |
| 1 | 17 | 0 | 9 | 0 |
| 1 | 28 | 6 | 18 | 0 |

# Skinny Recommended Breakfast Cereals

Look for cereals that contain 5 or more grams of fiber, 8 or fewer grams of sugar, and fewer than 200 calories per 1 cup serving. The following brands and varieties meet those specifications.

| | SERVING SIZE (cups) |
|---|---|
| General Mills Fiber One | ½ |
| Simply Fiber Cereal (Miracle Foods) | 1 |
| General Mills Fiber One Honey Clusters | 1¼ |
| Kellogg's All Bran Extra Fiber | ½ |
| Kashi GoLEAN | ¾ |
| Uncle Sam Cereal | 1 |
| Kellogg's All-Bran | ½ |
| Post 100% Bran | ⅓ |
| Kashi Good Friends | ¾ |
| Post Spoon Size Shredded Wheat | 1 |
| General Mills Wheat Chex | 1 |
| Kellogg's All-Bran Complete Wheat Flakes | ¾ |
| Post Bran Flakes | ¾ |
| Quaker Crunchy Corn Bran | ¾ |
| Kashi Heart to Heart | ¾ |
| Nature's Path Organic Shredded Heritage Bites | 1 |

| Calories | Fiber (g) | Protein (g) | Carbs (g) | Sugars (g) |
|---|---|---|---|---|
| 60 | 14 | 2 | 24 | 0 |
| 100 | 13 | 4 | 31 | 0 |
| 170 | 14 | 3 | 47 | 5 |
| 50 | 13 | 3 | 20 | 0 |
| 120 | 10 | 8 | 28 | 7 |
| 190 | 10 | 7 | 38 | 0 |
| 80 | 8 | 4 | 24 | 0 |
| 80 | 8 | 4 | 23 | 7 |
| 90 | 8 | 3 | 24 | 6 |
| 170 | 6 | 6 | 40 | 0 |
| 180 | 5 | 5 | 40 | 5 |
| 90 | 5 | 3 | 24 | 6 |
| 100 | 5 | 2 | 23 | 6 |
| 90 | 5 | 2 | 23 | 6 |
| 110 | 5 | 4 | 25 | 5 |
| 120 | 5 | 4 | 24 | 6 |

## Glycemic Loads of Common Foods

Glycemic load is a measure of how carbohydrate foods affect blood sugar. Whenever possible, opt for low-GL foods. Note the portion size of any food on the list. If you eat double the size, then double the GL. Also keep in mind that *Skinny* eating involves much more than a food's GL. I've seen some diets that claim you can have mashed potatoes—just add cream to them to slow the absorption of starch. This very well may reduce the GL of the meal, but it increases the calorie density, making the potatoes just as fattening if not more so. The same goes for French fries. Because of their high fat content, they are actually low in GL, but that doesn't mean they are not fattening. They contain so many calories in such a compact amount of space that it's nearly impossible to stop eating them before you've overeaten.

## The Skinny Foods List

Skinny foods are whole foods that are low in both glycemic load (GL) and calorie density. GL is the amount of carbohydrate in a portion of a food multiplied by its glycemic index (a measure of how that food affects blood sugar). Calorie density is a measure of the number of calories in a certain weight of food. It is usually measured in calories per gram. In my opinion, the higher the calorie density and the higher the glycemic load, the more "fattening" the food.

Whenever possible:

- Opt for foods with a GL of 9 or less; the lower the better.
- Note the portion size of any food on the list. If you eat double the size, then double the GL. The calorie density, on the other hand, doesn't change with portion size. This is important with certain foods like pasta, where the usual portion is bigger than the amount on the chart.
- Choose fruits, vegetables, dairy products, and soups with a calorie density of 0.6 or less, grain-based foods with a calorie density of 1.5 or less, and meats of 4 or less.
- Choose whole foods whenever possible.

Once you've lost weight and are maintaining, if want to have a food that's not a Skinny choice, have half the usual portion.

GL Key
1–9: low GL
10–19: medium GL
20+: high GL

Calorie Density Key
0.6 or less: very low
0.6 to 1.5: low
1.5 to 4: medium
4+: high

## Bread and Crackers

Serving size: 1 slice of bread or 1 ounce of crackers

| Food | Glycemic Load | Calorie Density | Is it a whole food? | Is it a Skinny choice? |
|------|---------------|-----------------|---------------------|------------------------|
| Whole-grain bread (100%) | 5 | 2.6 | Yes | In phase 2 |
| Pumpernickel bread | 5 | 2.5 | Yes | In phase 2 |
| Tortilla, 6-inch (white, wheat, or corn) | 5 | 3.1 | No | No |
| 9-grain bread | 6 | 2.6 | Yes | In phase 2 |
| Sourdough rye bread | 6 | 2.5 | Yes | In phase 2 |
| Sourdough whole-wheat bread | 6 | 2.5 | Yes | In phase 2 |
| Soda crackers (6 crackers) | 9 | 4.2 | No | No |
| Melba toast | 10 | 3.9 | No | No |

| Food | Glycemic Load | Calorie Density | Is it a whole food? | Is it a Skinny choice? |
|---|---|---|---|---|
| Pita bread, refined | 10 | 2.7 | No | No |
| White bread | 10 | 2.9 | No | No |
| Hamburger bun | 12 | 2.7 | No | No |
| White bagel | 40 | 2.5 | No | No |

## Grains and Rice

Serving size: ⅓ cup rice and other grains, ½ cup couscous

| Food | Glycemic Load | Calorie Density | Is it a whole food? | Is it a Skinny choice? |
|---|---|---|---|---|
| Brown rice | 6 | 1.1 | Yes | Yes |
| Barley | 7 | 1.2 | Yes | Yes |
| Bulgur | 8 | 0.8 | Yes | Yes |
| Long-grain white rice | 8 | 1.2 | No | Yes |
| Couscous | 11 | 1.1 | No | No |
| Jasmine rice | 15 | 1.3 | No | No |
| Instant rice | 16 | 1.3 | No | No |

## Pasta

Serving size: ⅓ cup

| Food | Glycemic Load | Calorie Density | Is it a whole food? | Is it a Skinny choice? |
|---|---|---|---|---|
| Egg noodles | 5 | 1.3 | No | No |
| Fettuccine | 5 | 1.3 | No | No |
| Spaghetti, refined | 5 | 1.3 | No | No |
| Spaghetti, whole-wheat | 5 | 1.3 | Yes | With dinner, as your starch side dish |
| Instant noodles | 6 | 1.3 | No | No |
| Rice noodles | 6 | 1 | No | No |
| Capellini | 7 | 1.3 | No | No |
| Linguine vermicelli | 7 | 1.3 | No | No |
| Cheese tortellini | 8 | 3 | No | No |
| Macaroni and cheese | 10 | 3.7 | No | No |

# Cereals

Serving size: varies

| Food | Glycemic Load | Calorie Density | Is it a whole food? | Is it a Skinny choice? |
|---|---|---|---|---|
| All-Bran, ½ cup | 5 | 2.6 | Yes | In phase 2 |
| Raisin Bran, ⅓ cup | 8 | 3.3 | No | No |
| Weetabix, 1 biscuit | 8 | 3.7 | No | No |
| Just Right, fruit & nut, ½ cup | 9 | 3.7 | No | No |
| Oatmeal, slow-cooked, ½ cup | 9 | 3.3 | Yes | In phase 2 |
| Quick Oats, ⅔ cup | 9 | 3.7 | No | No |
| Cheerios, ⅔ cup | 10 | 3.6 | No | No |
| Life Cereal, ½ cup | 10 | 3.7 | No | No |
| Mini-Wheats, ½ cup | 10 | 3.5 | No | No |
| Special K, ½ cup | 10 | 3.7 | No | No |
| Froot Loops, ⅔ cups | 11 | 3.9 | No | No |
| Golden Grahams, ½ cup | 11 | 4 | No | No |

| Food | Glycemic Load | Calorie Density | Is it a whole food? | Is it a Skinny choice? |
|------|---------------|-----------------|---------------------|------------------------|
| Corn Flakes, 2/3 cup | 12 | 3.8 | No | No |
| Wheaties, 2/3 cup | 12 | 3.6 | No | No |
| Rice Krispies, 2/3 cup | 13 | 3.8 | No | No |
| Shredded Wheat | 13 | 3.4 | No | No |

## Vegetables

Serving size: varies

| Food | Glycemic Load | Calorie Density | Is it a whole food? | Is it a Skinny choice? |
|------|---------------|-----------------|---------------------|------------------------|
| Bean sprouts, ¾ cup | 0 | 0.19 | Yes | Yes |
| Broccoli, ¾ cup | 0 | 0.34 | Yes | Yes |
| Brussels sprouts, ¾ cup | 0 | 0.43 | Yes | Yes |
| Celery, 2 stalks | 0 | 0.16 | Yes | Yes |
| Bell peppers, ¾ cup | 0 | 0.31 | Yes | Yes |
| Spinach, ¾ cup raw | 0 | 0.23 | Yes | Yes |
| Zucchini, ¾ cup | 0 | 0.21 | Yes | Yes |

| Food | Glycemic Load | Calorie Density | Is it a whole food? | Is it a Skinny choice? |
|---|---|---|---|---|
| Lettuce, 1 cup | 0 | 0.15 | Yes | Yes |
| Tomato, 1 medium | 1 | 0.84 | Yes | Yes |
| Green peas, 1/3 cup | 2 | 0.34 | Yes | Yes |
| Pumpkin, 1/2 cup | 2 | 0.24 | Yes | Yes |
| Tomato sauce, 1/2 cup | 3 | 0.24 | Yes | Yes |
| Baby carrots, 12 carrots | 4 | 0.35 | Yes | Yes |
| Beets, 1/2 cup | 5 | 0.44 | Yes | With dinner, as your starch side dish |
| Yams, 1/2 cup | 6 | 1.16 | Yes | With dinner, as your starch side dish |
| Tomato juice, 2 cups | 7 | 0.22 | No | No |
| Sweet potato, 2/3 potato | 9 | 0.92 | Yes | With dinner, as your starch side dish |
| Acorn squash, 1/2 cup | 10 | 0.56 | Yes | With dinner, as your starch side dish |
| Butternut squash, 1/2 cup | 10 | 0.4 | Yes | With dinner, as your starch side dish |

| Food | Glycemic Load | Calorie Density | Is it a whole food? | Is it a Skinny choice? |
|---|---|---|---|---|
| Sweet-corn kernels, ½ cup | 11 | 0.81 | Yes | With dinner, as your starch side dish |
| French fries, frozen, 12 fries | 12 | 3.16 | No | No |
| Baked potato, 1 medium | 14 | 0.93 | No | No |
| Mashed potatoes, ½ cup | 15 | 0.83 | No | No |
| Instant mashed potatoes, ½ cup | 17 | 1 | No | No |

## Beans and Legumes

Serving size: ½ cup

| Food | Glycemic Load | Calorie Density | Is it a whole food? | Is it a Skinny choice? |
|---|---|---|---|---|
| Soy beans | 1 | 1.4 | Yes | Yes |
| Black beans | 3 | 1.3 | Yes | Yes |
| Chick peas | 5 | 1.1 | Yes | Yes |
| Lima beans | 5 | .79 | Yes | Yes |
| Pinto beans | 6 | .86 | Yes | Yes |
| Split peas | 6 | 1.1 | Yes | Yes |
| Haricot and navy beans | 7 | 1.1 | Yes | Yes |

| Food | Glycemic Load | Calorie Density | Is it a whole food? | Is it a Skinny choice? |
|------|---------------|-----------------|---------------------|------------------------|
| Kidney beans | 7 | 0.84 | Yes | Yes |
| Baked beans | 9 | 1 | No | No |

## Soup

Serving size: varies

| Food | Glycemic Load | Calorie Density | Is it a whole food? | Is it a Skinny choice? |
|------|---------------|-----------------|---------------------|------------------------|
| Black bean, ½ cup | 5 | 0.46 | Yes | Yes |
| Split pea, ½ cup | 6 | 0.71 | Yes | Yes |
| Tomato, 1 cup | 6 | 0.6 | Yes | Yes |
| Minestrone, 1 cup | 7 | 0.53 | Yes | Yes |
| Lentil, 1 cup | 9 | 1.1 | Yes | Yes |

## Fruit

Serving size: varies

| Food | Glycemic Load | Calorie Density | Is it a whole food? | Is it a Skinny choice? |
|------|---------------|-----------------|---------------------|------------------------|
| Apple, 1 medium | 5 | 0.5 | Yes | Yes |
| Blueberries, 1 cup | 5 | 0.57 | Yes | Yes |
| Grapefruit, 1 whole | 5 | 0.32 | Yes | Yes |

| Food | Glycemic Load | Calorie Density | Is it a whole food? | Is it a Skinny choice? |
|---|---|---|---|---|
| Melon, 1 cup | 5 | 0.34 | Yes | Yes |
| Peach, 1 large | 5 | 0.39 | Yes | Yes |
| Raspberries, 1 cup | 5 | 0.52 | Yes | Yes |
| Strawberries, 20 medium or 1 cup frozen | 5 | 0.32 | Yes | Yes |
| Pear, 1 small | 6 | 0.58 | Yes | Yes |
| Pineapple, ½ cup | 6 | 0.5 | Yes | Yes |
| Prunes, 4 medium | 6 | 2.4 | Yes | Yes |
| Apricots, 4 medium | 7 | 0.48 | Yes | Yes |
| Cherries, 20 medium | 7 | 0.63 | Yes | Yes |
| Orange, 1 medium | 7 | 0.49 | Yes | Yes |
| Mango, ½ cup 3 medium | 8 | 0.65 | Yes | Yes |
| Plums, 3 medium | 8 | 0.46 | Yes | Yes |
| Peaches, in light syrup, 4 ounces | 9 | 0.42 | No | No |
| Banana, 1 small | 10 | 0.89 | Yes | No |
| Grapes, 25 small | 10 | 0.69 | Yes | No |

| Food | Glycemic Load | Calorie Density | Is it a whole food? | Is it a Skinny choice? |
|---|---|---|---|---|
| Kiwi fruit, 2 medium | 10 | 0.61 | Yes | No |
| Apple juice, 1¼ cup | 11 | 0.46 | No | No |
| Fruit cocktail, ¾ cup | 11 | 0.88 | No | No |
| Orange juice, 1¼ cup | 12 | 0.44 | No | No |
| Figs, dried, 2 | 13 | 2.4 | Yes | No |
| Lemonade, ¾ cup | 13 | 0.4 | No | No |
| Raisins, 3 tbsp | 13 | 3 | Yes | No |

## Miscellaneous

| Food | Glycemic Load | Calorie Density | Is it a whole food? | Is it a Skinny choice? |
|---|---|---|---|---|
| Peanuts, 1.75 ounces | 1 | 5.8 | Yes | Yes |
| 1% plain yogurt, ¾ cup | 3 | 0.6 | Yes | Yes |
| Skim milk, 1 cup | 4 | 0.3 | Yes | Yes |
| Jam, 1 tbsp | 7 | 2.7 | No | No |
| Oatmeal cookie, 1 ounce | 9 | 4.2 | No | No |

| Food | Glycemic Load | Calorie Density | Is it a whole food? | Is it a Skinny choice? |
|---|---|---|---|---|
| Popcorn, 3 cups popped | 10 | 3.8 | Yes | In phase 2 |
| Cheese pizza, 1 slice | 16 | 2.5 | No | No |
| Pretzels, 1 ounce | 16 | 3.7 | No | No |
| Tortilla chips, 1.75 ounces | 17 | 4.8 | No | No |
| Pancakes, 2 to 4 inches | 39 | 2.2 | No | No |

# Acknowledgments

Many people helped shape the ideas, words, and overall message that eventually became the pages of this book. I'm deeply grateful for the following:

- All of the patients who've been under my care during my more than twenty-year career. It's important to understand that I believe you. It was your bravery and continued effort in the face of a demoralizing illness that keeps me continually searching for more effective weight-loss solutions.
- The many researchers whose studies helped me put the puzzle pieces together. Especially, I'm indebted to Dr. Rudy Leibel of Columbia University, who got me started on this path and who has been instrumental in developing many of the fundamental concepts that have changed the field. The same goes for Dr. Mike Rosenbaum of Columbia and his work on the physiology of the reduced state. Dr. George Blackburn from Harvard University encouraged me to work on obesity in the late 1980s when everyone else thought I was crazy. The tough

mentoring from Jules Hirsch from Rockefeller University forced me to develop a sharply honed argument. I've repeatedly used and cited Dr. Barbara Rolls's elegant work on eating and the concept of "calorie density"; Harvard's Dr. David Ludwig's work on the impact of glycemic index on eating, metabolism, and weight loss; the University of Washington's Dr. Michael Schwartz's work on neuroendocrine aspects of weight regulation; and Dr. Uberto Pagotto and Dr. Vincenzo Demarzo's work on the endocannabinoid system. Dr. Judy Korner, from Columbia, is a collaborator, a joke teller, and an excellent researcher who helped me focus many of these ideas. Dr. Tom Wadden from the University of Pennsylvania is a giant in the field of clinical obesity research. You're a great role model. Dr. Karen Segal also helped me so much over the years. There are many other colleagues in the field from whom I have learned so much: Apovian, Eckel, Fujioka, Hill, Jensen, Kushner, Klein, Kaplan, and others. I must also thank the dedicated staff of the Comprehensive Weight Control Program, including Dr. Jon Waitman, Dr. Ileana Vargas, and Judy Townsend, PA, MPH.

- My wife, Jane. You not only kept the office running smoothly and made sure I stayed on schedule with writing the book, you also generously offered to be the model in the photos that appear in this book.

- Heather Bainbridge, Dr. Kathy Isoldi, and Janet Feinstein, all dietitians at the Comprehensive Weight Control Program. Thank you for your valuable insights as well as helping assemble the menu plans, some of the recipes, and the nutritional advice in this book.

- My coauthor, Alisa Bowman, for downloading everything I know about weight loss from my brain to yours, organizing it, and finding an exciting way to present it.

- David Vigliano and Michael Harriot. You believed in the need for this book long before I did. Thank you for persuading me to write it.

- Stacy Creamer and everyone at Broadway Books, for enthusiastically believing in this project from the beginning and especially for embracing the unpopular message that weight problems are not a matter of personal weakness or willpower, but rather a symptom of a biological problem that needs a more in-depth approach than seen before.

- Beth Bischoff. No one shoots better fitness photos than you.
- Christopher J. Daly, Master Trainer, Medical Exercise Specialist. Your professionalism and attention to detail produced the fitness photos in record time.
- Jennifer Kushnier, for developing some of the recipes that are included in this book.
- Suzanne Wright and Lupe Minero for putting up with my ranting and raving.
- My children, Allison and Louis, for generally putting up with me.
- My parents, Theresa and Albert, for their support.

# Selected Bibliography

Chapter 1

Adam TC, Jocken J, Westerterp-Plantenga M. Decreased glucagon-like peptide 1 release after weight loss in overweight/obese subjects. *Obesity.* 2005; 13:710–716.

Aronne LJ, Isoldi KK. Cannabinoid-1 receptor blockade in cardiometabolic risk reduction: efficacy. *American Journal of Cardiology.* 2007 Dec 17;100(12A): 18P–26P.

Bakhøj S, Flint A, Holst JJ, Tetens I. Lower glucose-dependent insulinotropic polypeptide (GIP) response but similar glucagon-like peptide 1 (GLP-1), glycaemic, and insulinaemic response to ancient wheat compared to modern wheat depends on processing." *European Journal of Clinical Nutrition.* 2003;57: 1254–1261.

Blundell JE, Stubbs RJ, Golding C, Croden F, Alam R, Whybrow S, Le Noury J, Lawton CL. Resistance and susceptibility to weight gain: individual variability in response to a high-fat diet. *Physiology & Behavior.* 2005;86:614–622.

Campos M, Aguilera C, Canete R, Gil A. Ghrelin: a hormone regulating food intake and energy homeostasis. *British Journal of Nutrition.* 2006;96:201–226.

Cummings D. Ghrelin and the short- and long-term regulation of appetite and body weight. *Physiology & Behavior.* 2006;89:71–84.

Enroiri P, Evans A, Sinnayah P, Cowley M. Leptin resistance and obesity. *Obesity.* 2006;14:254S–258S.

Flier J. Regulating energy balance: the substrate strikes back. *Science.* 2006; 312:861–864.

Frezza E, Wachtel M, Chiriva-Internati M. The multiple faces of glucagon-like peptide-1—obesity, appetite, and stress: what is next? *Digestive Diseases & Sciences.* 2007;52:643–649.

Getty-Kaushik L, Song D, Boylan M, Corkey B, Wilfe M. Glucose-dependent insulinotropic polypeptide modulates adipocyte lipolysis and reesterification. *Obesity.* 2006;14:1124–1131.

Kirkham TC, Tucci SA. Endocannabinoids in appetite control and the treatment of obesity. *CNS & Neurological Disorders—Drug Targets.* 2006;5:275–292.

Klok MD, Jakobsdottir S, Drent ML. Appetite regulatory peptides. *Obesity Reviews.* 2007;8:21–34.

Korner J, Aronne LJ. The emerging science of body weight regulation and its impact on obesity treatment. *Journal of Clinical Investigation.* 2003;111: 565–570.

Kunos G. Understanding metabolic homeostasis and imbalance: what is the role of the endocannabinoid system? *American Journal of Medicine.* 2007; 120(suppl 1):S18–S24.

Levin B. The obesity epidemic: metabolic imprinting on genetically susceptible neural circuits. *Obesity.* 2000;8:342–347.

Matias I, Di Marzo V. Endocannabinoids and the control of energy balance. *Trends in Endocrinology & Metabolism.* 2007;18(1):27–37.

Meyers M, Patti E, Leshan R. Hitting the target: leptin and perinatal nutrition in the predisposition to obesity. *Endocrinology.* 2005;146:4209–4210.

Morton G. Hypothalamic leptin regulation of energy homeostasis and glucose metabolism. *Journal of Physiology.* 2007;583(pt 2):437–443.

Morton GJ, Cummings DE, Baskin DG, Barsh GS, Schwartz MW. Central nervous system control of food intake and body weight. *Nature.* 2006;443: 289–295.

Power C, Jefferis B. Fetal environment and subsequent obesity: a study of maternal smoking. *International Journal of Epidemiology.* 2002;31:413–419.

Reed DR, Lawler MP, Tordoff MG. Reduced body weight is a common effect of gene knockout in mice. *BMC Genetics.* 2008;9:4.

Shankar K, Harrell AM, Liu X, Gilchrist JM, Ronis MJ, Badger TM. Maternal obesity at conception programs obesity in the offspring. *American Journal of Physiology: Regulatory, Integrative & Comparative Physiology.* 2008;294:R528–R538.

Shimizu H, Oh-I S, Okada S, Mori M. Leptin resistance and obesity. *Endocrine Journal.* 2007;54:17–26.

Snethen JA, Hewitt JB, Goretzke M. Childhood obesity: the infancy connection. *Journal of Obstetric Gynecological & Neonatal Nursing.* 2007;36: 501–510.

Stephenson T, Symonds ME. Maternal nutrition as a determinant of birth weight. *Archives of Disease in Childhood: Fetal Neonatal Edition.* 2002;86: F4–F6.

Stock S, Leichner P, Wong A, Ghatei M, Kieffer T, Bloom S, Chanoine JP. Ghrelin, peptide YY, glucose-dependent insulinotropic polypeptide, and hunger responses to a mixed meal in anorexic, obese, and control female adolescents. *Journal of Clinical Endocrinology & Metabolism.* 2005;90:2161–2168.

Sturm R. Increases in morbid obesity in the USA: 2000–2005. *Public Health.* 2007;121:492–496.

Wang GJ, Volkow ND, Logan J, Pappas NR, Wong CT, Zhu W, Netusil N, Fowler JS. Brain dopamine and obesity. *Lancet.* 2001;357:354–357.

Wisse B, Kim F, Schwartz M. An integrative view of obesity. *Science.* 2007;318:928–929.

Wu Q, Suzuki M. Parental obesity and overweight affect the body-fat accumulation in the offspring: the possible effect of a high-fat diet through epigenetic inheritance. *Obesity Reviews.* 2006;7:201–208.

Young A. Obesity: a peptide YY-deficient, but not peptide YY-resistant, state. *Endocrinology.* 2006;147:1–2.

## Chapter 2

Albuquerque KT, Sardinha FL, Telles MM, Watanabe RL, Nascimento CM, Tavares do Carmo MG, Ribeiro EB. Intake of trans fatty acid-rich hydrogenated fat during pregnancy and lactation inhibits the hypophagic effect of central insulin in the adult offspring. *Nutrition.* 2006;22:820–829.

Anderson G, Catherine N, Woodend D, Wolever T. Inverse association between the effect of carbohydrates on blood glucose and subsequent short-term food intake in young men. *American Journal of Clinical Nutrition.* 2002;76: 1023–1030.

Avena N. Examining the addictive-like properties of binge eating using an animal model of sugar dependence. *Experimental & Clinical Psychopharmacology.* 2007;15:481–491.

Avena N, Long K, Hoebel B. Sugar dependent rats show enhanced responding for sugar after abstinence: evidence of a sugar deprivation effect. *Psychology & Behavior.* 2005;84:359–362.

Avena N, Rada P, Hoebel B. Evidence for sugar addiction: behavioral and neurochemical effects of intermittent, excessive sugar intake. *Neuroscience & Biobehavioral Reviews.* 2008;32:20–39.

Bensaïd A, Tomé D, Gietzen D, Even P, Morens C, Gausseres N, Fromentin G. Protein is more potent than carbohydrate for reducing appetite in rats. *Physiology & Behavior.* 2002;75:577–582.

Blundell JE, Stubbs RJ, Golding C, Croden F, Alam R, Whybrow S, Le Noury J, Lawton CL. Resistance and susceptibility to weight gain: individual variability in response to a high-fat diet. *Physiology & Behavior.* 2005;86:614–622.

Colantuoni C, Rada P, McCarthy J, Patten C, Avena N, Chadeayne A, Hoebel B. Evidence that intermittent, excessive sugar intake causes endogenous opioid dependence. *Obesity.* 2002;10:478–488.

Colantuoni C, Schwenker J, McCarthy J, Rada P, Ladenheim B, Cadet J, Schwartz G, Moran T, Hoebel B. Excessive sugar intake alters binding to dopamine and mu-opioid receptors in the brain. *NeuroReport.* 2001;12:3549–3552.

Corcoran MP, Lamon-Fava S, Fielding RA. Skeletal muscle lipid deposition and insulin resistance: effect of dietary fatty acids and exercise. *American Journal of Clinical Nutrition.* 2007;85:662–677.

Cotton JR, Burkey VJ, Weststrate JA, Blundell JE. Dietary fat and appetite: similarities and differences in the satiating effect of meals supplemented with either fat or carbohydrate. *Journal of Human Nutrition & Diet.* 2007;20:186–199.

Davidson TL, Swithers SE. A Pavlovian approach to the problem of obesity. *International Journal of Obesity.* 2004;28:933–935.

De Souza CT, Araujo EP, Bordin S, Ashimine R, Zollner RL, Boschero AC, Saad MJ. Consumption of a fat-rich diet activates a proinflammatory response and induces insulin resistance in the hypothalamus. *Endocrinology.* 2005; 146:4192–4199.

Ebbeling CB, Leidig MM, Feldman HA, Lovesky MM, Ludwig DS. Effects of a low-glycemic load vs. low-fat diet in obese young adults: a randomized trial. *Journal of the American Medical Association.* 2007;297:2092–2102.

Ibrahim A, Natrajan S, Ghafoorunissa R. Dietary trans-fatty acids alter adipocyte plasma membrane fatty acid composition and insulin sensitivity in rats. *Metabolism.* 2005;54:240–246.

Kwun IS, Cho YE, Lomeda RA, Kwon ST, Kim Y, Beattie JH. Marginal zinc deficiency in rats decreases leptin expression independently of food intake and corticotrophin-releasing hormone in relation to food intake. *British Journal of Nutrition.* 2007;98:485–489.

Leahy KE, Birch LL, Rolls BJ. Reducing energy density of an entree decreases children's energy intake at lunch. *Journal of the American Dietetic Association.* 2008;108:41–48.

Ledford H. Excessive fat intake can throw out the body clock. *Nature.* 2007; 450:141.

Ledikwe JH, Ello-Martin J, Pelkman CL, Birch LL, Mannino ML, Rolls BJ. A reliable, valid questionnaire indicates that preference for dietary fat declines when following a reduced-fat diet. *Appetite.* 2007;49:74–83.

Lenoir M, Serre F, Cantin L, Ahmed SH. Intense sweetness surpasses cocaine reward. *PLoS ONE*. 2007;2:e698.

Little TJ, Horowitz M, Feinle-Bisset C. Modulation by high-fat diets of gastrointestinal function and hormones associated with the regulation of energy intake: implications for the pathophysiology of obesity. *American Journal of Clinical Nutrition*. 2006;86:531–541.

Liu C, Grigson PS. Brief access to sweets protect against relapse to cocaine seeking. *Brain Research*. 2005;1049:128–131.

Major GC, Doucet E, Jacqmain M, St-Onge M, Bouchard C, Tremblay A. Multivitamin and dietary supplements, body weight and appetite: results from a cross-sectional and a randomized double-blind placebo-controlled study. *British Journal of Nutrition*. 2008;99:1157–1167.

Mazlan N, Horgan G, Whybrow S, Stubbs J. Effects of increasing increments of fat- and sugar-rich snacks in the diet on energy and macronutrient intake in lean and overweight men. *British Journal of Nutrition*. 2006;96:596–606.

Nachtigal MC, Patterson RE, Stratton KL, Adams LA, Shattuck AL, White E. Dietary supplements and weight control in a middle-age population. *Journal of Alternative & Complementary Medicine*. 2005;11:909–915.

Pereira MA, Swain J, Goldfine AB, Rifai N, Ludwig DS. Effects of low-glycemic load diet on resting energy expenditure and heart disease risk factors during weight loss. *Journal of the American Medical Association*. 2004;292:2482–2490.

Rada P, Avena NM, Hoebel B. Daily bingeing on sugar repeatedly releases dopamine in the accumbens shell. *Neuroscience*. 2005;134:737–744.

Raeseland JE, Anderson SA, Solvoll K, Hjermann I, Urdal P, Holme I, Drevon CA. Effect of long-term changes in diet and exercise on plasma leptin concentrations. *American Journal of Clinical Nutrition*. 2001;73:240–245.

Tzima N, Pitsavos C, Panagiotakos D, Skoumas D, Zampelas A, Chrysohoou C, Stefanadis C. Mediterranean diet and insulin sensitivity, lipid profile and blood pressure levels in overweight and obese people; the Attica study. *Lipids in Health & Heart Disease*. 2007;6:22

Vozzo R, Wittert G, Cocchiaro C, Tan WC, Mudge J, Fraser R, Chapman I. Similar effects of foods high in protein, carbohydrate and fat on subsequent spontaneous food intake in healthy individuals. *Appetite*. 2003;40:101–107.

Westerterp-Plantenga MS, Smeets A, Lejeuune MP. Sensory and gastrointestinal satiety effects of capsaicin on food intake. *International Journal of Obesity*. 2005;29:682–688.

Wideman CH, Nadzam GR, Murphy HM. Implications of an animal model of sugar addiction, withdrawal and relapse for human health. *Nutritional Neuroscience*. 2005;8:269–276.

Yoshioka M, Imanaga M, Ueyama H, Yamane M, Kubo Y, Boivin A, St-Amand J, Tanaka H, Kiyonaga A. Maximum tolerable dose of red pepper decreases fat intake independently of spicy sensation in the mouth. *British Journal of Nutrition.* 2004;91:991–995.

## Chapter 3

Nilsson AC, Ostman EM, Holst JJ, Björck IM. Including indigestible carbohydrates in the evening meal of healthy subjects improves glucose tolerance, lowers inflammatory markers, and increases satiety after a subsequent standardized breakfast. *Journal of Nutrition.* 2008;138:732–739.

## Chapter 4

Araya H, Hills J, Alvina M, Vera G. Short-term satiety in preschool children: a comparison between a high protein meal and a high complex carbohydrate meal. *International Journal of Food Science & Nutrition.* 2002;51:119–124.

Arumugam V, Lee JS, Nowak JK, Pohle RJ, Nyrop JE, Leddy JJ, Pelkman CL. A high-glycemic meal pattern elicited increased subjective appetite sensations in overweight and obese women. *Appetite.* 2008;50:215–222.

Barkoukis H, Marchetti CM, Nolan B, Sistrun SN, Krishnan RK, Kirwan JP. A high glycemic meal suppresses the postprandial leptin response in normal healthy adults. *Annals of Nutrition & Metabolism.* 2007;51:512–518.

Bazzano LA, Song Y, Bubes V, Good CK, Manson JE, Liu S. Dietary intake of whole and refined grain breakfast cereals and weight gain in men. *Obesity.* 2005;13:1952–1960.

Blom W, Lluch A, Stafleu A, Vinoy S, Holst J, Schaafsma G, Hendriks H. Effect of high-protein breakfast on postprandial ghrelin response. *American Journal of the College of Nutrition.* 2006;83:211–220.

Buyken AE, Trauner K, Günther AL, Kroke A, Remer T. Breakfast glycemic index affects subsequent daily energy intake in free-living healthy children. *American Journal of Clinical Nutrition.* 2007;86:980–987.

Childs JL, Yates MD, Drake MA. Sensory properties of meal replacement bars and beverages made from whey and soy proteins. *Journal of Food Science.* 2007;72:S425–S434.

Croezen S, Visscher TL, Ter Bogt NC, Veling ML, Haveman-Nies A. Skipping breakfast, alcohol consumption and physical inactivity as risk factors for overweight and obesity in adolescents: results of the E-MOVO project. *European Journal of Clinical Nutrition.* 2007 Nov 28. [Epub ahead of print]

Farshchi HR, Taylor MA, Macdonald IA. Deleterious effects of omitting breakfast on insulin sensitivity and fasting lipid profiles in healthy lean women. *American Journal of Clinical Nutrition.* 2005;81:388–396.

Fischer K, Colombani PC, Langhans W, Wenk C. Carbohydrate to protein ratio in food and cognitive performance in the morning. *Physiology & Behavior.* 2002;75:411–423.

Fischer K, Colombani PC, Wenk C. Metabolic and cognitive coefficients in the development of hunger sensations after pure macronutrient ingestion in the morning. *Appetite.* 2004;42:49–61.

Frecka JM, Mattes RD. Possible entrainment of ghrelin to habitual meal patterns in humans. *American Journal of Physiology: Gastrointestinal & Liver Physiology.* 2008;294:G699–G707.

Henry CJ, Lightowler HJ, Strik CM. Effects of long-term intervention with low- and high-glycaemic-index breakfasts on food intake in children aged 8–11 years. *British Journal of Nutrition.* 2007;98:636–640.

Hlebowicz J, Wickenberg J, Fahlström R, Björgell O, Almér LO, Darwiche G. Effect of commercial breakfast fibre cereals compared with corn flakes on postprandial blood glucose, gastric emptying and satiety in healthy subjects: a randomized blinded crossover trial. *Nutrition Journal.* 2007;6:22.

Holt SH, Delargy HJ, Lawton CL, Blundell JE. The effects of high-carbohydrate vs. high-fat breakfasts on feelings of fullness and alertness, and subsequent food intake. *International Journal of Food Science & Nutrition.* 1999;50:13–28.

Holzmeister LA. *The Ultimate Calorie, Carb & Fat Gram Counter.* Alexandria, Va: Small Steps Press; 2006.

Ingwersen J, Defeyter MA, Kennedy DO, Wesnes KA, Scholey AB. A low glycaemic index breakfast cereal preferentially prevents children's cognitive performance from declining throughout the morning. *Appetite.* 2007;49:240–244.

Khan A, Safdar M, Ali Khan MM, Khattak KN, Anderson RA. Cinnamon improves glucose and lipids of people with type 2 diabetes. *Diabetes Care.* 2003;26:3215–3218.

Kim HH, Lee S, Jeon TY, Son HC, Kim YJ, Sim MS. Post-prandial plasma ghrelin levels in people with different breakfast hours. *European Journal of Clinical Nutrition.* 2004;58:692–695.

Johnston CS, Day CS, Swan PD. Postprandial thermogenesis is increased 100% on a high-protein, low-fat diet versus a high-carbohydrate, low-fat diet in healthy, young women. *Journal of the American College of Nutrition.* 2002;21:55–61.

Ludwig DS, Majzoub JA, Al-Zahrani A, Dallal GE, Blanco I, Roberts SB. High glycemic index foods, overeating, and obesity. *Pediatrics.* 1999;103:E26.

Nilsson AC, Ostman EM, Granfeldt Y, Björck IM. Effect of cereal test breakfasts differing in glycemic index and content of indigestible carbohydrates on daylong glucose tolerance in healthy subjects. *American Journal of Clinical Nutrition.* 2008;87:645–654.

Nilsson AC, Ostman EM, Holst JJ, Björck IM. Including indigestible carbohydrates in the evening meal of healthy subjects improves glucose tolerance, lowers inflammatory markers, and increases satiety after a subsequent standardized breakfast. *Journal of Nutrition.* 2008;138:732–739.

Nilsson A, Radeborg K, Björck I. Effects of differences in postprandial glycaemia on cognitive functions in healthy middle-aged subjects. *European Journal of Clinical Nutrition*. 2007 Sep 12. [Epub ahead of print]

Purslow LR, Sandhu MS, Forouhi N, Young EH, Luben RN, Welch AA, Khaw KT, Bingham SA, Wareham NJ. Energy intake at breakfast and weight change: prospective study of 6,764 middle-aged men and women. *American Journal of Epidemiology*. 2008;167:188–192.

Smeets AJ, Westerterp-Plantenga MS. Acute effects on metabolism and appetite profile of one meal difference in the lower range of meal frequency. *British Journal of Nutrition*. 2008;99:1316–1321.

van der Heijden AA, Hu FB, Rimm EB, van Dam RM. A prospective study of breakfast consumption and weight gain among U.S. men. *Obesity*. 2007;15: 2463–2469.

Vander Wal JS, Marth JM, Khosla P, Jen KL, Dhurandhar NV. Short-term effect of eggs on satiety in overweight and obese subjects. *Journal of the American College of Nutrition*. 2005;24:510–515.

Warren JM, Henry CJ, Simonite V. Low glycemic index breakfasts and reduced food intake in preadolescent children. *Pediatrics*. 2003;112:e414.

## Chapter 5

Ello-Martin JA, Roe LS, Ledikwe JH, Beach AM, Rolls BJ. Dietary energy density in the treatment of obesity. *American Journal of Clinical Nutrition*. 2007;85:1465–1477.

Johnston CS, Buller AJ. Vinegar and peanut products as complementary foods to reduce post prandial glycemia. *Journal of the American Dietetic Association*. 2005;105:1939–1942.

Leeman M, Ostman E, Björck J. Vinegar dressing and cold storage of potatoes lowers postprandial glycaemic and insulinaemic responses in healthy subjects. *European Journal of Clinical Nutrition*. 2005;59:1266–1271.

Ostman E, Granfeldt Y, Persson L, Björck I. Vinegar supplementation lowers glucose and insulin responses and increases satiety after a bread meal in healthy subjects. *European Journal of Clinical Nutrition*. 2005;59:983–988.

Rolls BJ, Bell EA, Thorwart ML. Water incorporated into a food but not served with a food decreases energy intake in lean women. *American Journal of Clinical Nutrition*. 1999;70:448–455.

Rolls BJ, Roe LS, Meengs JS. Salad and satiety: energy density and portion size of a first-course salad affect energy intake at lunch. *Journal of the American Dietetic Association*. 2004;104:1570–1576.

Rolls BJ, Roe LS, Meengs JS, Wall DE. Increasing the portion size of a sandwich increases energy intake. *Journal of the American Dietetic Association*. 2004;104: 367–372.

Smeets AJ, Westerterp-Plantenga MS. Acute effects on metabolism and appetite profile of one meal difference in the lower range of meal frequency. *British Journal of Nutrition*. 2008;99:1316–1321.

Westerterp-Plantenga MS. Protein intake and energy balance. *Regulatory Peptides*. 2008 Mar 25. [Epub ahead of print]

Westerterp-Plantenga MS, Smeets A, Lejeune MP. Sensory and gastrointestinal satiety effects of capsaicin on food intake. *International Journal of Obesity*. 2005; 29:682–688.

Yoshioka M, Imanaga M, Ueyama H, Yamane M, Kubo Y, Boivin A, St-Amand J, Tanaka H, Kiyonaga A. Maximum tolerable dose of red pepper decreases fat intake independently of spicy sensation in the mouth. *British Journal of Nutrition*. 2004;91:991–995.

## Chapter 6

Flood JE, Rolls BJ. Soup preloads in a variety of forms reduce meal energy intake. *Appetite*. 2007;49:626–634.

Levitsky DA, Halbmaier CA, Mrdjenovic G. The freshman weight gain: a model for the study of the epidemic of obesity. *International Journal of Obesity Related Metabolism Disorders*. 2004;28:1435–1442.

Mazlan N, Horgan G, Whybrow S, Stubbs J. Effects of increasing increments of fat- and sugar-rich snacks in the diet on energy and macronutrient intake in lean and overweight men. *British Journal of Nutrition*. 2006;96:596–606.

Osterholt KM, Roe LS, Rolls BJ. Incorporation of air into a snack food reduces energy intake. *Appetite*. 2007;48:351–358.

Read D, van Leeuwen B. Predicting hunger: the effects of appetite and delay on choice. *Organizational Behavior & Human Decision Processes*. 1998;76: 189–205.

Rolls BJ, Roe LS, Kral TV, Meengs JS, Wall DE. Increasing the portion size of a packaged snack increases energy intake in men and women. *Appetite*. 2004;42:63–69.

Rolls BJ, Roe LS, Meengs JS. The effect of large portion sizes on energy intake is sustained for 11 days. *Obesity*. 2007;15:1535–1543.

Wansink B, Kim J. Bad popcorn in big buckets: portion size can influence intake as much as taste. *Journal of Nutrition Education & Behavior*. 2005;37: 242–245.

## Chapter 7

Bellissimo N, Pencharz PB, Thomas SG, Anderson GH. Effect of television viewing at mealtime on food intake after a glucose preload in boys. *Pediatric Research*. 2007;61:745–749.

de Castro JM. The time of day and the proportions of macronutrients eaten are related to total daily food intake. *British Journal of Nutrition*. 2007;98: 1077–1083

de Castro JM. The time of day of food intake influences overall intake in humans. *Journal of Nutrition*. 2004;134:104–111.

Flood JE, Rolls BJ. Soup preloads in a variety of forms reduces meal energy intake. *Appetite*. 2007;49:626–634.

Keim NL, Van Loan MD, Horn WF, Barbieri TF, Mayclin PL. Weight loss is greater with consumption of large morning meals and fat-free mass is preserved with large evening meals in women on a controlled weight reduction regimen. *Journal of Nutrition*. 1997;127:75–82.

Mattes R. Soup and satiety. *Physiology & Behavior*. 2005;83:739–747.

Rolls BJ, Bell EA, Thorwart ML. Water incorporated into a food but not served with a food decreases energy intake in lean women. *American Journal of Clinical Nutrition*. 1999;70:448–455.

Rolls BJ, Roe LS, Meengs JS. The effect of large portion sizes on energy intake is sustained for 11 days. *Obesity*. 2007;15:1525–1543.

Rolls BJ, Roe LS, Meengs JS. Reductions in portion size and energy density of foods are additive and lead to sustained decreases in energy intake. *American Journal of Clinical Nutrition*. 2006;83:11–17.

Westerterp-Plantenga MS, Smeets A, Lejeune MP. Sensory and gastrointestinal satiety effects of capsaicin on food intake. *International Journal of Obesity*. 2005;29:682–688.

Yoshioka M, Imanaga M, Ueyama H, Yamane M, Kubo Y, Boivin A, St-Amand J, Tanaka H, Kiyonaga A. Maximum tolerable dose of red pepper decreases fat intake independently of spicy sensation in the mouth. *British Journal of Nutrition*. 2004;91:991–995.

## Chapter 8

Almiron-Roig E, Drewnowski A. Hunger, thirst, and energy intakes following consumption of caloric beverages. *Physiology & Behavior*. 2003;79:767–773.

Appleton KM, Blundell JE. Habitual high and low consumers of artificially-sweetened beverages: effects of sweet taste and energy on short-term appetite. *Physiology & Behavior*. 2007;92:479–486.

Appleton KM, Rogers PJ, Blundell JE. Effects of a sweet and a nonsweet lunch on short-term appetite: differences in female high and low consumers of sweet/low-energy beverages. *Journal of Human Nutrition & Dietetics*. 2004;17: 425–434.

Bell EA, Roe LS, Rolls BJ. Sensory-specific satiety is affected more by volume than by energy content of a liquid food. *Physiology & Behavior*. 2003;78: 593–600.

Bellisle F, Drewnowski A. Intense sweeteners, energy intake and the control of body weight. *European Journal of Clinical Nutrition.* 2007;61:691–700.

Black RM, Leiter LA, Anderson GH. Consuming aspartame with and without taste: differential effects on appetite and food intake of young adult males. *Physiology & Behavior.* 1993;53:459–466.

Bowen J, Noakes M, Clifton PM. Appetite hormones and energy intake in obese men after consumption of fructose, glucose and whey protein beverages. *International Journal of Obesity.* 2007;31:1696–1703.

Caton SJ, Ball M, Ahern A, Hetherington M. Dose-dependent effects of alcohol on appetite and food intake. *Physiology & Behavior.* 2004;81:51–58.

DellaValle DM, Roe LS, Rolls BJ. Does the consumption of caloric and noncaloric beverages with a meal affect energy intake? *Appetite.* 2005;44:187–193.

Elfhag K, Tynelius P, Rasmussen F. Sugar-sweetened and artificially sweetened soft drinks in association to restrained, external and emotional eating. *Physiology & Behavior.* 2007;91:191–195.

Harper A, James A, Flint A, Astrup A. Increased satiety after intake of a chocolate milk drink compared with a carbonated beverage, but no difference in subsequent ad libitum lunch intake. *British Journal of Nutrition.* 2007;97: 579–583.

Holt SH, Sandona N, Brand-Miller JC. The effects of sugar-free vs sugar-rich beverages on feelings of fullness and subsequent food intake. *International Journal of Food Science & Nutrition.* 2000;51:59–71.

Jones KL, O'Donovan D, Horowitz M, Russo A, Lei Y, Hausken T. Effects of posture on gastric emptying, transpyloric flow, and hunger after a glucose drink in healthy humans. *Digestive Diseases & Sciences.* 2006;51:1331–1338.

Lavin JH, French SJ, Read NW. The effect of sucrose- and aspartame-sweetened drinks on energy intake, hunger and food choice of female, moderately restrained eaters. *International Journal of Obesity Related Metabolism Disorders.* 1997;21:37–42.

Mattes R. Soup and satiety. *Physiology & Behavior.* 2005;83:730–747.

Mattes RD, Rothacker D. Beverage viscosity is inversely related to postprandial hunger in humans. *Physiology & Behavior.* 2001;74:551–557.

Melanson KJ, Zukley L, Lowndes J, Nguyen V, Angelopoulos TJ, Rippe JM. Effects of high-fructose corn syrup and sucrose consumption on circulating glucose, insulin, leptin, and ghrelin and on appetite in normal-weight women. *Nutrition.* 2007;23:103–112.

Mourao DM, Bressan J, Campbell WW, Mattes RD. Effects of food form on appetite and energy intake in lean and obese young adults. *International Journal of Obesity.* 2007;31:1688–1695.

Rolls BJ, Bell EA, Thorwart ML. Water incorporated into a food but not served with a food decreases energy intake in lean women. *American Journal of Clinical Nutrition.* 1999;70:448–455.

Rolls BJ, Kim S, Fedoroff IC. Effects of drinks sweetened with sucrose or aspartame on hunger, thirst and food intake in men. *Physiology & Behavior.* 1990; 48:19–26.

Soenen S, Westerterp-Plantenga MS. No differences in satiety or energy intake after high-fructose corn syrup, sucrose, or milk preloads. *American Journal of Clinical Nutrition.* 2007;86:1586–1594.

Tsuchiya A, Almiron-Roig E, Lluch A, Guyonnet D, Drewnowski A. Higher satiety ratings following yogurt consumption relative to fruit drink or dairy fruit drink. *Journal of the American Dietetic Association.* 2006;106:550–557.

Van Walleghen EL, Orr JS, Gentile CL, Davy BM. Pre-meal water consumption reduces meal energy intake in older but not younger subjects. *Obesity.* 2007; 15:93–99.

Wannamethee SG, Field A, Colditz G, Rimm E. Alcohol intake and 8-year weight gain in women: a prospective study. *Obesity.* 2004;12:1386–1396.

Zijlstra N, Mars M, de Wijk RA, Westerterp-Plantenga MS, de Graaf C. The effect of viscosity on ad libitum food intake. *International Journal of Obesity.* 2007;32:676–683.

## Chapter 9

Ara I, Perez-Gomez J, Vicente-Rodriguez G, Chavarren J, Dorado C, Calbet JA. Serum free testosterone, leptin and soluble leptin receptor changes in a 6-week strength-training programme. *British Journal of Nutrition.* 2006;96:1053–1059.

Ashworth NL, Chad KE, Harrison EL, Reeder BA, Marshall SC. Home versus center based physical activity programs in older adults. *Cochrane Database of Systematic Reviews.* 2005; Jan 25(1):CD00417.

Blumenthal JA, Babyak M, Moore KA, Craighead WE, Herman S, Khatri P, Waugh R, Napolitano MA, Forman LM, Appelbaum M, Dorauswamy PM, Krishnam R. Effects of exercise training on older patients with major depression. *Archives of Internal Medicine.* 1999;159:2349–2356.

Blundell JE, Stubbs RJ, Hughes DA, Whybrow S, King NA. Cross talk between physical activity and appetite control: does physical activity stimulate appetite? *Proceedings of the Nutrition Society.* 2003;62:651–661.

Bravata DM, Smith-Spangler C, Sundaram V, Gienger AL, Lin N, Lewis R, Stave CD, Olkin I, Sirard JR. Using pedometers to increase physical activity and improve health: a systematic review. *Journal of the American Medical Association.* 2007;298:2296–2304.

Burns N, Finucane FM, Hatunic M, Gilman M, Murphy M, Gasparro D, Maru A, Gastaldelli A, Nolan JJ. Early onset type 2 diabetes in obese white subjects is characterized by a marked defect in beta cell insulin secretion, severe insulin resistance, and a lack of response to aerobic exercise training. *Diabetologia.* 2007;50:1500–1508.

Candow DG, Burke DG. Effect of short-term equal-volume resistance training with different workout frequency on muscle mass and strength in untrained men and women. *Journal of Strength Conditioning Research.* 2007;21: 204–207.

Cox KL, Burke V, Gorely TJ, Beilin LJ, Puddy IB. Controlled comparison of retention and adherence in home vs. center initiated exercise interventions in women ages 40–65 years: the S.W.E.A.T. study (Sedentary Women Exercise Adherence Trial). *Preventative Medicine.* 2003;36:17–29.

Dietrich A, McDaniel WF. Endocannabinoids and exercise. *British Journal of Sports Medicine.* 2004;38:536–541.

Doucet E, Imbeault P, St-Pierre S, Alméras N, Mauriège P, Després JP, Bouchard C, Tremblay A. Greater than predicted decrease in energy expenditure during exercise after body weight loss in obese men. *Clinical Science.* 2003; 105:89–95.

Eisenmann J, DuBose K, Donnelly J. Fatness, fitness, and insulin sensitivity among 7 to 9 year old children. *Obesity.* 2007;15:2135–2144.

Erdmann J, Tahbaz R, Lippl F, Wagenpfeil S, Schusdziarra V. Plasma ghrelin levels during exercise—Effects of intensity and duration. *Regulatory Peptides.* 2007;143:127–135.

Granner M, Sharpe P, Hutto B, Wilcox S, Addy C. Perceived individual social and environmental factors for physical activity and walking. *Journal of Physical Activity & Health.* 2007;4:278–293.

Hamilton MT, Hamilton DG, Zderic TW. Role of low energy expenditure and sitting in obesity, metabolic syndrome, type 2 diabetes, and cardiovascular disease. *Diabetes.* 2007;56:2655–2667.

Harris C, DeBeliso MA, Spitzer-Gibson TA, Adams KJ. The effect of resistance-training intensity on strength-gain response in the older adult. *Journal of Strength Conditioning Research.* 2004;18:833–838.

Hassmen P, Koivula N, Uutela A. Physical exercise and psychological well-being: a population study in Finland. *Preventative Medicine.* 2000;30:17–25.

Janssen I, Katzmarzyk PT, Ross R, Leon AS, Skinner JS, Rao DC, Wilmore JH, Rankinen T, Bouchard C. Fitness alters the associations of BMI and waist circumference with total and abdominal fat. *Obesity.* 2004;12:525–537.

Kodama S, Shu M, Saito K, Murakami H, Tanaka K, Kuno S, Ajisaka R, Sone Y, Onitake F, Takahashi A, Shimano H, Kondo K, Yamada N, Sone H. Even low intensity and low volume exercise training may improve insulin resistance in the elderly. *Internal Medicine.* 2007;46:1071–1077.

Miyashita M, Tokuyama K. Moderate exercise reduces serum triacylglycerol concentrations but does not affect pre-heparin lipoprotein lipase concentrations after a moderate-fat meal in young men. *British Journal of Nutrition.* 2008;99: 1076–1082.

Munn J, Herbert RD, Hancock MJ, Gandevia SC. Resistance training for strength: effect of number of sets and contraction speed. *Medicine & Science in Sports & Exercise.* 2005;37:1622–1626.

Reed JA, Phillips DA. Relationships between physical activity and the proximity of exercise facilities and home exercise equipment used by undergraduate university students. *Journal of the American College of Health.* 2005;53:285–290.

Richardson CR, Mehari KS, McIntyre LG, Janney AW, Fortlage LA, Sen A, Strecher VJ, Piette JD. A randomized trial comparing structures and lifestyle goals in an internet-mediated walking program for people with type 2 diabetes. *International Journal of Behavioral Nutrition & Physical Activity.* 2007;4:59.

Ronnestad BR, Egeland W, Kvamme NH, Refsnes PE, Kadi F, Raastad T. Dissimilar effects of one and three set strength training on strength and muscle mass gains in upper and lower body in untrained subjects. *Journal of Strength Conditioning Research.* 2007;21:157–163.

Sallis JF, Hovell MF, Hofstetter CR, Elder JP, Hackley M, Caspersen CJ, Powell KE. Distance between homes and exercise facilities related to frequency of exercise among San Diego residents. *Public Health Reports.* 1990;105:179–185.

Shaw K, Gennat H, O'Rourke P, Del Mar C. Exercise for overweight or obesity. *Cochrane Database Systematic Reviews.* 2006;Oct 18(4):CD003817.

Szeinbach S, Seoane-Vazquez E, Parekh A, Herderick M. Dispensing errors in community pharmacy: perceived influence of sociotechnical factors. *International Journal for Quality Health Care.* 2007;19:203–209.

White LJ, Dressendorfer RH, Holland E, McCoy SC, Ferguson MA. Increased caloric intake soon after exercise in cold water. *International Journal of Sport Nutrition & Exercise Metabolism.* 2005;15:38–47.

## Chapter 10

Aronne LJ. Therapeutic options for modifying cardiometabolic risk factors. *American Journal of Medicine.* 2007;120(3A):S26–S34.

Atkinson G, Davenne D. Relationships between sleep, physical activity and human health. *Physiology & Behavior.* 2007;90:229–235.

Gangwisch JE, Malaspina D, Bodon-Albala B, Heymsfield SB. Inadequate sleep as a risk factor for obesity: analysis of NHANES. *Sleep.* 2005;28:1289–1296.

Patel SR, Malhotra A, White DP, Gottlieb DJ, Hu FB. Association between reduced sleep and weight gain in women. *American Journal of Epidemiology.* 2006;164:947–954.

Ramakrishnan K, Scheid DC. Treatment options for insomnia. *American Family Physician.* 2007;76:517–526.

Reilly T, Waterhouse J. Jet lag and air travel: implications for performance. *Clinical Sports Medicine.* 2005;24:367–380.

Schwartz JR, Roth T. Shift work sleep disorder. *Drugs.* 2006;66:2357–2370.

Vorona RD, Winn MP, Babineau TW, Eng BP, Feldman HR, Ware CW. Overweight and obese patients in a primary care population report less sleep than patients with normal body mass index. *Archives of Internal Medicine.* 2005;165:25–30.

Waterhouse J. Jet-lag and shift work: circadian rhythms. *Journal of the Royal Society of Medicine.* 1999;92:398–401.

Waterhouse J, Reilly T, Atkinson G, Edwards B. Jet lag: trends and coping strategies. *Lancet.* 2007;369:1117–1129.

## Chapter 11

Klem ML, Wing RR, Lang W, McGuire MT, Hill JO. Does weight loss maintenance become easier over time? *Obesity.* 2000;8:438–444.

Levitsky D. The non-regulation of food intake in humans: hope for reversing the epidemic of obesity. *Physiology & Behavior.* 2005;86:623–632.

Phelan S, Hill JO, Lang W, Dibello JR, Wing RR. Recovery from relapse among successful weight maintainers. *American Journal of Clinical Nutrition.* 2003; 78:1079–1084.

Phelan S, Wyatt HR, Hill JO, Wing RR. Are the eating and exercise habits of successful weight losers changing? *Obesity.* 2006;14:710–716.

Raynor DA, Phelan S, Hill JO, Wing RR. Television viewing and long-term weight maintenance: results from the national weight control registry. *Obesity.* 2006;14:1816–1823.

# Index

## Subjects

abdominal fat, 14, 18
acanthosis nigricans, 14
accredited obesity surgery programs, 152
Acomplia, 147–48
Adipex, 147
adiponectin, 17, 41
alcohol
  appetite and, 40, 92, 94, 160
  sleep problems and, 140, 141
allergy medications, 143–144
Allī, 146–47
American College of Surgeons, 152
antidepressants, 144, 150
antioxidants, 85
appetite, 3–20
  alcohol and, 40, 92, 94, 160
  breakfast's effect on, 56–58
  genetic influence, 10
  naturally skinny people, 4–6
  order of eating and, 31–32, 41, 71, 91, 160
  psychological vs. biological factors, 4–5, 6–7

refined starch and, 92–93
sleep problems and, 138–39
sweetened beverages and, 106–7
  *See also* fullness and fullness resistance; hunger
appetizers
  dinner, 46, 91–92, 93
  lunch, 44, 73
artificial sweeteners, 26–27, 106–7

beans, calorie density and glycemic loads, 215–16
beer, 40
  *See also* alcohol
beverage makeover, 103–9
  how to do it, 107–8
  making it happen, 108–10
  why it works, 104–6
beverages, 40
  alcoholic, 40, 92, 94, 140, 141, 160
  fruit juice, 65–66, 68, 109, 218
  sweetened beverages, 103–9
bitter orange, 151

rebound hunger, 22, 23, 25, 27,
106–7, 161
weight-loss maintenance and, 159
*See also* fullness and fullness
resistance
hunger hormones, 7, 16–18
cortisol, 18, 139
endocannabinoids (ECs), 16–17, 19,
147–48
*See also* ghrelin
hydrogenated fats, 25–26
*See also* dietary fat

implanted fullness stimulators, 154
Indian restaurants, 96
infants, factors influencing infants'
weight outcomes, 10, 11
inflammation, 13, 23
insomnia, 141
insulin, 14–15
ECs and, 17
exercise and, 112, 132
leptin resistance and, 19–20
sleep problems and, 139
weight-loss medications and, 146,
148
yo-yo dieting and, 38
insulin resistance, 14–15
blood sugar, carbohydrates and, 14, 23
cortisol and, 18
dietary fats and, 26
leptin and, 13, 14, 15
skipping breakfast and, 57
insulin sensitivity
diabetes medications and, 148–49
gastric bypass surgery and, 153
insulin therapy, alternative medication,
149
Italian restaurants, 78–79, 96–97

Japanese restaurants, 78, 97
jet lag, 142–43
journals. *See* food diary; lifestyle log
juice, 65–66, 68, 109, 218

Kosher salt, 192

lactic acidosis, 149
lap band surgery, 152
late-night snacks, 57, 67, 82–83

LDL, 57
weight-loss medications and, 146
lean protein, 24–25, 27, 28
*See also* protein
legumes, 24
calorie density, 215–16
glycemic loads, 215–16
Leibel, Rudolph, 12, 112
leptin and leptin resistance, 11,
12–14, 15
body heat/metabolism and, 17, 112,
157
carbohydrates and, 23
ECs and, 16
inflammation and, 13
insulin and, 19–20
insulin resistance and, 13, 14, 15
leptin levels in infants, 11
protein and, 28
saturated fats and, 25
sleep deprivation and, 138–39
triglycerides and, 13
weight loss and, 18–19, 112, 156
lifestyle activity, 36, 116–17, 132, 164
lifestyle log, 35–37, 48
lipodystrophy, 14
liquids, 30, 68, 105–6
liquid calories, 27–28, 104–5
liquid diets, 60–61
*See also* beverage makeover; beverages
liver weight, 162–63
low-calorie foods, 28–29
low-fat diets, 24–25
lunch makeover, 34, 69–79
bread and sandwiches, 49, 72, 74, 75
eating-out advice, 77–79
how to do it, 70–75
making it happen, 76–77
Phase 1 lunch options, 44–45
Phase 2 lunch options, 49
why it works, 69–70

main courses
dinner, 46, 92, 93
lunch, 45, 74
main dish recipes, 172–82
maintaining weight loss, 34, 38,
155–65
keeping a maintenance graph,
158–59

maintaining weight loss (*cont.*)
  losing weight you regain, 163–65
  maintenance diet, 42–43, 47–49,
    156
  stopping the yo-yo cycle, 161–63
  tips for, 157–61
  your maintenance weight, 155–57
marijuana, 16
McDonald's, 79, 98
meal replacement shakes, 109, 163
  *See also* protein shakes
meat, 24–25, 29, 161
medications, 143–51
  alternatives to medications that cause
    weight gain, 148–50
  sleep aids, 140, 143–44
  as weight-loss barrier, 143–46
  weight-loss medications, 146–48,
    150–51
  what not to take, 150–51
  *See also specific medications*
Meridia, 146
metabolism
  body heat and, 17
  breakfast and, 57
  insulin resistance and, 15
  low-GL diet and, 23
  muscle mass and, 112, 113
  overmetabolism, 13
  protein and, 28
  time of day and, 90
  weight loss and, 10, 18–19, 112–13,
    155, 156, 157
metformin, 148–49
Mexican restaurants, 78, 97
migraine medications, 144, 149–50
milk, 218
  on cereal, 63–64
mood disorder medications, 144, 150
movement makeover, 34, 111–33
  advanced program, 125–31
  beginner's program, 119–21
  how to do it, 115–18
  intermediate program, 121–25
  making it happen, 131–33
  why it works, 112–14
  *See also* exercise
multivitamins, 29
muscle cell function, 13, 15, 17
  weight loss plateau and, 18

muscle mass
  metabolism and, 112, 113
  *See also* strength training
mustard, 195

night shift work, 142
nuts, 81–82, 85, 88, 218

oatmeal, 47, 63–64
obesity genes, 9, 11
obesity statistics, 13
obesity surgery
  choosing a surgeon, 151–52
  surgery options, 152–54
  when to consider, 151
orlistat, 146–47
overeating
  at or after dinner, 100–102
  cheat nights or meals, 42
  food hangovers, 57, 162
  getting back on track after, 57, 102,
    161–62
  overmetabolism and, 13
  rebound hunger, 22, 23, 25, 27,
    106–7, 161
overmetabolism, 13

pasta, 31
  calorie density, 211
  glycemic loads, 211
  *See also* starch, starchy foods
peanut butter, 65
peanuts, 218
pedometers, 131
peptide YY, 16
Phase 1 plan, 42–47, 156
Phase 2 plan
  menus, 47–49
  switching to, 42–43, 156
phen-fen, 147
phentermine, 147
plate size, 40
portion sizes, 39
  dinner, 89, 90–91
  fattening foods, 91
  snacks, 87
  starchy foods, 41
pramlintide, 149
pregnancy, factors influencing babies'
    weight outcomes, 10, 11

# Recipes

# About the Author

DR. LOUIS ARONNE is an internationally recognized expert in weight control who has directed the Comprehensive Weight Control Program at New York–Presbyterian Hospital/Weill Cornell Medical Center since 1986. Dr. Aronne has been president of the Obesity Society and is a fellow of the American College of Physicians. He edited the National Institutes of Health *Practical Guide to the Identification, Evaluation, and Treatment of Overweight and Obesity in Adults* and has authored more than forty papers and book chapters on obesity. Dr. Aronne was one of the founding hosts of the TV Food Network, cohosting more than 650 episodes of *Getting Healthy,* a nightly call-in show covering a broad variety of topics in health, nutrition, and medicine. He has made dozens of appearances on *Late Night with David Letterman* and the *Late Show with David Letterman* since the 1980s, and is perhaps best known for diagnosing Dave's heart problem in 2000. Since 2001 he has been ranked annually in Castle Connolly's *Top Doctors: New York Metro Area* directory as a specialist in obesity, diabetes, and internal medicine. Dr. Aronne founded the Cardiometabolic Support Network (cmsnonline.com), a unique treatment program to improve the quality of life for patients suffering from obesity and obesity-related illnesses. He lives in Greenwich, Connecticut.